What is Health?

What is Health?

Ruth Cross

polity

The right of Ruth Cross to be identified as Author of this Work has been asserted in accordance with the UK Copyright, Designs and Patents Act 1988.

First published in 2024 by Polity Press

Polity Press
65 Bridge Street
Cambridge CB2 1UR, UK

Polity Press
111 River Street
Hoboken, NJ 07030, USA

ISBN-13: 978-1-5095-5648-9
ISBN-13: 978-1-5095-5649-6(pb)

A catalogue record for this book is available from the British Library.

Library of Congress Control Number: 2023950666

Typeset in 10.5 on 12pt Sabon
by Fakenham Prepress Solutions, Fakenham, Norfolk NR21 8NL
Printed and bound in Great Britain by CPI Group (UK) Ltd, Croydon

The publisher has used its best endeavours to ensure that the URLs for external websites referred to in this book are correct and active at the time of going to press. However, the publisher has no responsibility for the websites and can make no guarantee that a site will remain live or that the content is or will remain appropriate.

Every effort has been made to trace all copyright holders, but if any have been overlooked the publisher will be pleased to include any necessary credits in any subsequent reprint or edition.

For further information on Polity, visit our website:
politybooks.com

Contents

Detailed Contents

Dedicated to my nieces, nephews and goddaughters.
You bring me so much happiness, thank you. I hope you
live healthy, happy lives – whatever that looks like to each
of you.
Love you all, always and forever.

Acknowledgements

I would like to acknowledge the contribution of the following people and extend my sincere gratitude to them.

Polity Press for supporting the development of this book from start to finish, particularly Jonathan Skerrett for his instrumental advice throughout the process, and Karina Jákupsdóttir for her patience in working together to finalize the book cover.

The students I work with, from whom I learn something new every day.

The anonymous reviewers who took the time to read through draft chapters and provide valuable and constructive comments. Your contribution has made this a more rounded book. I hope I have done your insights justice.

MAC, thank you for everything.

Introduction

For those working in health, health promotion or any health-related field, understanding what health *is* (what it means to people) is crucial for implementing effective policy and practice. Often, however, the students I work with on the programmes I teach have a relatively narrow understanding of health. Their viewpoints then change significantly as they are exposed to, and engage with, different ideas and perspectives.

This book came into being because I wanted to write a more in-depth piece of work about what health *is*, having already written several introductory chapters on this subject in books on health studies, health promotion and public health. A few thousand words cannot do justice to the complexity of health. This book does not do full justice to it either, but it does provide greater scope to consider what health is in more detail and to better explore its complexities and nuances. As such it includes discussion about many aspects of the subject, including different definitions, perspectives, dimensions and models of health; experiences of health; and determinants of health. It also discusses health as happiness and as well-being, as well as considering what creates health. The final chapter focuses on planetary health. A range of disciplines are drawn upon throughout the book, taking in ideas from sociology, psychology and economics.

There are several key themes within the book. At the outset it is important to note that the book has been written from the perspective that health is (largely) socially constructed, although it is also recognized that there is a physical dimension to health experience. In addition, positivist and social constructionist notions of health interact and influence each other and cannot be easily disentangled. Research, evidence and lay and Indigenous perspectives from around the world are drawn upon throughout the book to bring the discussion to life and give context. Lay perspectives are particularly important from a social constructionist perspective, and they can help bring some of the theoretical discussion into sharper focus.

The scene for the rest of the book is set in Chapter 1, which considers the question 'what is health?', acknowledging at the outset that the subject is complex and contested. The chapter starts by outlining why it is necessary to think about health in detail and to consider what health is. It examines different definitions of health, including the World Health Organization's classic definition. The chapter introduces different philosophies of health and ideas of what it means to be 'healthy', drawing attention to the complicated and debated nature of health and differing lived experiences. It explores the social construction of health and highlights the importance of lay perspectives. More critical debates are also introduced in this chapter, in particular those around health as a social construct and as a moral phenomenon.

Chapter 2 explores the nature of health as multi-dimensional. In this chapter several different dimensions of health will be considered, each in turn. At the outset it is acknowledged that this is a highly theoretical, conceptual approach to take, since each dimension is not entirely discrete and different dimensions of health will overlap, intersect and interact to some extent. Nevertheless, the following dimensions are considered: physical health, mental health, spiritual health, emotional health, social health and societal health. Finally, the notion of holistic health is outlined and discussed as a means of bringing the different dimensions together as well as offering a new perspective on health which considers the 'whole person'. Lay perspectives on health are intertwined throughout the discussion, drawing on research and evidence from around the world and taking into account the multitude of factors that impact on people's ideas about health (for example, culture, age and gender).

The theoretical basis for thinking about health is provided in Chapter 3. This chapter starts with an exploration of Lalonde's health field concept. Several other models are then introduced, discussed and critiqued. These include the biomedical model of health, the social model of health, the biopsychosocial model of health (Sarafino and Smith, 2022) and a 'working model of health' that brings together aspects of the preceding models (Green et al., 2019). Each model is described and outlined in detail. The chapter then moves on to consider non-western models of health as rooted within Indigenous understandings of health and well-being. These are considered in general terms before looking in some detail at Indigenous concepts of health in Māori populations in New Zealand and Indigenous communities in Canada.

Chapter 4 considers what determines health. It starts by exploring what is meant by the term 'determinants of health' and then moves on to introduce two models of social determinants: Dahlgren and Whitehead's (1991) classic 'rainbow' model and the more contemporary framework provided by the Commission on the Social Determinants of Health (Solar and Irwin, 2010). The social determinants of health are discussed in relation to these two models. This includes consideration of structural determinants such as social class, gender and commercial determinants of health. The chapter examines health inequalities and inequity and draws on a range of international research to illustrate how health experience is inconsistent between, and within, countries in our modern world. This includes some discussion about responsibility for health, as well as issues of structure and agency. The seminal work of Sir Michael Marmot and his team is considered in some detail in this chapter, which ends with some final thoughts on how the social determinants of health might be tackled in order to create fairer health outcomes for all.

The idea of health as *well-being* is explored in Chapter 5, starting with an exploration of different definitions and concepts of well-being. It discusses Grant et al.'s (2007) three core elements of well-being – psychological, physical and social – as well as some other theoretical contributions, including that offered by Martin Seligman. The chapter draws on a range of research about well-being and health using lay perspectives as a basis for the discussion. The challenges of measuring well-being are considered, taking into account how ideas about it vary according to different social factors such as culture and race/ethnicity. The chapter includes an overview of the Geneva Charter for Well-being and ends with a brief discussion about quality of life.

In the past two decades happiness has become more generally linked to health and health experience in the broader literature. Some people would even argue that to be happy is to be healthy. Happiness indices now offer a way of measuring quality of life outside of economic means. Chapter 6 explores what happiness *is* and how it relates to concepts of what it means to be healthy. Happiness is considered firstly at the individual level and then at societal level. Happiness research is drawn upon throughout the chapter, and reference is made to relevant theoretical constructs of happiness. There is also some discussion of how happiness can be measured and achieved, drawing on narratives of health and happiness from the wider literature. The chapter concludes with a case study of happiness, health and social media.

Chapter 7 concerns the question of what makes people healthy. While the previous chapters consider several different perspectives on what health is and what determines it, in this chapter we turn our attention to what *creates* health. As well as giving due attention to action on the social determinants of health this chapter focuses more heavily on salutogenic perspectives and asset-based approaches to creating health. It begins with a brief discussion of policy approaches to tackling the social determinants of health, then moves on to Aaron Antonovsky's theory of salutogenesis. The discussion draws upon global research and evidence from the wider literature about the effectiveness of salutogenic approaches to health, and suggests how these might be maximized for health gain, before moving on to consider asset-based approaches.

Planetary health affects everyone. The health of our planet and our own health are intricately connected. Chapter 8, the final chapter, locates the discussion about human health within the context of planetary health. It draws attention to the critical issues of our time, including climate change, overpopulation and threats of extinction. Discussing the concept of ecological health, it introduces some relevant theoretical constructs that seek to describe and explain the complex interactions between human health and the health of our planet. The chapter draws on Indigenous concepts that view human health as inextricably linked to planetary health and discusses how both might be addressed for the benefit of all. Finally, it discusses the future of human health over the next few decades in the light of current knowledge about human and planetary health, recognizing some of the challenges that are faced and how they might be overcome.

In each chapter you will find the following features to enable your understanding:

- A set of aims outlining what the chapter will do.
- Opportunities to 'pause for reflection', which will give you the chance to think about and reflect on the chapter contents in more detail.
- A case study designed to bring aspects of the discussion in the chapter to life.
- A summary section outlining the main points of the chapter.
- A suggestion for further reading. This may be a paper, a book chapter or even a book.

I hope you enjoy reading this book as much as I have enjoyed researching and writing it.

1
What is Health?

Chapter aims

- To consider health as complex and contested
- To examine different definitions of health, including the World Health Organization's classic definition
- To explore health as socially constructed
- To highlight the importance of lay perspectives and lived experiences of health

Introduction

This chapter considers the question 'what is health?' as a broad introduction the rest of the book. It provides the foundation for the subsequent discussions in the following chapters and sets the context for discovering the nature of health. The chapter starts by outlining why it is necessary to think about health in detail and to consider what health *is*, acknowledging from the outset that ideas about it are complex and contested. Different definitions and concepts of health from the wider literature are introduced and discussed, including the 'classic' definition offered by the World Health Organization. The chapter introduces different philosophies of health and ideas of what it means to be 'healthy', drawing attention to the complicated and debated nature of health and differing lived experiences. More critical debates about health are also introduced, such as health conceived as a social construct and as a moral phenomenon. Finally, the importance of lay perspectives on health will be considered, as a basis for this being a key theme throughout the book.

The importance of health

Why is health important? Perhaps you could take a few minutes to think about this. Is health important to you? If so, why? Most people, when asked what is important to them or what they value most, will mention health at some point. For some people health is *the* most important thing, viewed as an integral or essential part of life. After all, being healthy generally means experiencing life in a more meaningful, enjoyable way as well as enabling us to do what we desire. Health, however, is a nebulous concept, and what it means to one person is likely to be different to what it means to another (Tapper, 2021).

Health: complex and contested

The notion of health, then, is highly complex, and there are many ways in which it can be defined, understood and experienced (Cross, 2020). Although the word 'health' is frequently used, its meaning is often taken for granted or there is assumed to be a shared understanding about what it is. However, if you ask any number of people what health means to them you are likely to get different answers, although there may be some common themes in the responses. What we understand health to be is influenced by many factors, including where we live, our age, our gender, our health experience and status, the era in which we were born and so on.

One of the simplest ways of thinking about health is a dichotomous one – health can be viewed either positively or negatively (Green et al., 2019). Positive ideas about health tend to emphasize aspects such as well-being, happiness and holism. Such ideas encompass very broad perspectives on health and what it means to be healthy, taking into account the many dimensions of health (see the further discussion of this in Chapter 2). On the other hand, negative definitions of health tend to focus on not being ill, and the absence of disease or disability. Negative definitions therefore tend to be narrower, more focused on our physiology (the physical body), and rooted in the (bio)medical model of health that promotes scientific understandings about what health is. However, these definitions tend to overlook subjective perspectives on health: people's everyday experiences, under-standings and realities of health (Cross et al., 2017). So, health can also be viewed as socially constructed. We will consider this in more detail later in this chapter.

Health may also be seen as a value, as a right or as a responsibility. Mahatma Gandhi highlighted health as a value when he said in 1948: 'It is health that is real wealth and not pieces of gold and silver' (cited in Oleribe et al., 2018: npn), emphasizing the importance of health compared to being rich. Many people will put a high value on health when asked about the things that are important to them; however, health may not always be a priority, depending on the circumstances of a person's life. The pursuit of health for its own sake will often come second to other more pressing concerns.

There is ongoing debate about health as a right and health as a responsibility. Many would argue that everyone has a right to health and, indeed, this is enshrined in the Universal Declaration of Human Rights (1948), which states in Article 25 that 'everyone has a right to a standard of living adequate for the health and well-being of [themselves and their family], including food, clothing, housing and medical care and necessary social services, and the right to security in the event of unemployment, sickness, disability, widowhood, old age or other lack of livelihood in circumstances beyond [their] control'. Already we can see how this right to health encompasses many aspects of life. The right to health was recognized again in the 1966 International Covenant on

Economic, Social and Cultural Rights (WHO, 2008), and health has more recently been highlighted in Sustainable Development Goal 3: *Ensure healthy lives and promote well-being for all at all ages.*

Nampewo et al. (2022) contend that the right to health is one of the cornerstones for enhancing and improving overall well-being and human development, and that there are many different stakeholders who have a significant role to play in this, including individuals, states, corporations and institutions, as well as the international community. Nampewo et al. argue that everyone has a duty to play their part and that this implies a responsibility too. Health as a right is reflected in the Constitution of the World Health Organization, which states that 'the enjoyment of the highest attainable standard of health is one of the fundamental rights of every human being' (cited in WHO, 2008: 5), 'without distinction of race, religion, political belief, economic or social condition' (WHO, 2023: npn). As we have just seen, the right to health is also reinforced in Article 25 of the Universal Declaration of Human Rights in relation to the right to an adequate standard of living. Many of the other articles in that declaration are also directly or indirectly related to the right to health. Most people acknowledge that, for anyone to achieve health, basic human needs have to be met first, such as shelter, food and basic sanitation (Capone et al., 2018).

Health can also be understood in terms of consumption and as something that can be bought through either goods or services (Aggleton, 1990). The framing of health as a market or consumer need that requires services and products (pharmacological, technical, financial, etc.) is compelled by the (bio)medical model (see Chapter 3 for more detail). More recently, ideas about health have been influenced by social media, where there is a daily proliferation of posts about healthy eating and physical activity that emphasize the idea of health as a project, as something to be improved or acquired (Baker and Rojek, 2019). Such ideas also promote notions of health as consumption.

What 'being healthy' looks like might vary from person to person, too. Humanist perspectives on health emphasize our ability to adapt, cope and achieve our maximum potential whatever that might be, recognizing that not everyone can achieve the same end results (Morilla and del Palacio, 2016). Such perspectives link health directly to ideas about self-actualization, self-realization and self-fulfilment (Svalastog et al., 2017), another area where social media can play a key role.

Professional and lay understandings of health may differ or have similarities; however, there is good evidence to suggest that lay understandings of health are often complex and sophisticated (Cross, 2020). This is despite the fact that, as Green et al. (2019) argue, lay perspectives are often under-valued and seen to be illogical, unsound and inconsequential compared to so-called expert opinion. The complexities and sophistication of lay perspectives on health will become apparent when we return to them later in this chapter and throughout the book.

Definitions of health

As Angela Scriven (2017) argues, it is very hard to define health. In fact, finding a universally agreed definition would be impossible. Nevertheless, there are several different ways of defining health that can aid our understanding of what it is, and of how people experience and make sense of it. Definitions of health vary considerably dependent on a range of factors. Some definitions construe health as being an objective reality that can be assessed and measured (usually by establishing the absence of disease, illness, distress or injury). Such understandings are grounded in positivist ways of viewing the world which imply that there is an absolute truth that is discoverable. Definitions of health that centre on the absence of disease or illness reflect this type of worldview.

In contrast, other definitions consider the fact that health is a subjective experience and that understandings about what health *is* are not just rooted in our physical being but extend far beyond this. In this sense health is understood as being socially constructed, as socially, historically, culturally and temporally located (Warwick-Booth et al., 2021). We will explore the idea of health as a social construction in more detail later in this chapter. Suffice to say here that, as sociologist Mildred Blaxter (2010: 35) argues, 'health is not, in the minds of most people, a unitary concept. Health is multi-dimensional, and it is quite possible to have "good" health in one respect, but "bad" health in another.' For some people it is impossible to define health given that it is an abstract concept (Earle, 2007: 38), amorphous (Oleribe et al., 2018) and elusive (Johnson, 2007). However, others *have* tried to define it. Psychiatrist Norman Sartorius (2006: 662) notes three types of definition as follows:

1. Health as the absence of any disease or impairment
2. Health as a state that allows the individual to adequately cope with all demands of daily life (implying also the absence of disease and impairment), and
3. Health as a state of balance, an equilibrium that an individual has established within [themself] and between [themself] and [their] social and physical environment.

The first type of definition is quite narrow, restricting health to the physical or biological domain, but it sits well with an objective view of the world and might also be described as 'negative', since it is based on what health is *not*. Negative definitions of health do tend be narrower, more concerned with health as the absence of illness, and, unsurprisingly, more disease-oriented. Conversely, as noted earlier, positive definitions of health are broader, more concerned with health as well-being or as an asset (Warwick-Booth et al., 2021).

The second type of definition locates health at the individual level as well, but with more of an emphasis on functioning. The third type of definition, however, broadens the notion of health, moving beyond the individual (body) to encompass the wider environment. Notably, this type of definition reflects ideas about balance or equilibrium which are often found in lay understandings of health (Bishop and Yardley, 2010).

Definitions of health may focus on different *aspects* of health. Some (as in the second type of definition above) are concerned with health as the ability to function, to do the things we want to and get on with living (Warwick-Booth et al., 2021). Other definitions of health position it as a commodity, something that can be consumed, bought, sold, given or lost (Aggleton, 1990; Bambra et al., 2005). Humanist definitions of health cohere around ideas of being able to cope, adapt and achieve our greatest potential, expressed as self-actualization, self-fulfilment or self-realization (Svalastog et al., 2017). In keeping with this approach, David Seedhouse (2001: 8) defines health as the foundation for achievement, stating that a person's optimal health is 'equivalent to the set of conditions that enable a person to work to fulfil their realistic chosen and biological potentials'.

Stokes et al. (1982: 33) defined health as 'a state characterized by anatomic, physiologic and psychological integrity; an ability to perform personally valued family, work, and community roles; an ability to deal with physical, biologic, psychological, and social stress'. Oleribe et al. (2018) point out that this definition encompasses the notion of resilience, a concept that is often linked to mental health. Resilience is understood to be about our ability to cope with life's stressors and adapt to what life brings.

Warwick-Booth et al. (2021) highlight the fact that trying to produce a definition of health that suits everyone is very difficult as health is conceived of, experienced and influenced in so many different ways. In the same vein, Seedhouse (2001) argued that the question 'what is health?' is a philosophical one because competing and contrasting ideas about health exist. Viewing health in this way allows for an appreciation of its complexities and for different definitions and experiences of health to co-exist: as Wills (2023: 2) argues, health 'can embody a range of meanings, from the narrowly technical to the all-embracing moral or philosophical'.

Finally, as Scriven (2017) points out, it is important to appreciate that definitions of health change over time. They are constantly evolving as our understandings and experiences change too. How we define health will depend on many things, and, in that sense, health is highly subjective. Take, for example, our age. As we get older, we are more likely to consider health in terms of what we are still able to do, and in terms relative to our experiences of chronic illness – the chances of which increase with the years. Whether or not we are currently experiencing 'better' or 'worse' health will influence how we think about and define it (Tapper, 2021). Definitions of health have also changed over the course of human history as our knowledge of what causes and contributes to better health has developed. For example, before germs were discovered in the late nineteenth century, the cause of many infectious diseases was believed to be 'miasma' (literally: 'bad air'). Similarly, before the carcinogenic effects of cigarettes were known, smoking was promoted for medicinal purposes (Charlton, 2004). Advances in science, medicine and technology have affected ideas about what health is and what causes disease. They are likely to continue to do so. Before you read any further, take some time out to do Pause for Reflection 1.1.

Pause for Reflection 1.1

As pointed out above, definitions of health are not constant, and they change over time. Can you think of any examples of this? Use the internet to research ideas of health in a specific era (for example: medieval, pre-industrial, post-industrial). More recently, how did the COVID-19 pandemic change ideas about health and how to stay healthy?

The contribution of the World Health Organization

The World Health Organization has played an important role in the development of ideas about health. Many will be familiar with the classic definition of health offered by the WHO in its constitution: 'Health is a state of complete physical, mental and social well-being and not merely the absence of disease and infirmity' (WHO, 1948, cited in WHO, 2006a). This definition has a lot going for it. It is broad. It is positively framed, marking a move away from understanding health in a narrow, medical, disease-oriented way. It recognizes that health is more than simply not being ill. It takes into account mental and social health, and it brings in ideas about well-being. It locates health in subjective experience

(McDonald, 2023). Notably, it promotes a holistic view of health as well.

This definition has stood the test of time quite well over the seventy-five years or so it has been around, but it has also come under fire for several reasons too. It is viewed by many as being unrealistic, impossible to attain and even utopian in nature (Huber, 2011; Lucas and Lloyd, 2005; Tapper, 2021). Such criticisms centre on the fact that no one could describe themselves as being healthy with this definition as their point of reference. It has also been criticized for not taking into account other dimensions of health. Whilst it references physical, mental and social health, it does not include other recognized dimensions such as emotional, spiritual or environmental health for example. Some people, such as Francesco Chirico (2016), have called for the WHO to revise its definition of health to include the spiritual dimension, but this has not yet happened. More than twenty years ago epidemiologist Rodolfo Saracci (1997: 1409) highlighted several shortcomings with the definition, stating that it was of no practical use and that it seemed to 'more accurately define happiness than health'. Sartorius (2006: 662), among others, has pointed to a major problem with the definition in its failure to recognize that health can 'co-exist with the presence of a disease or impairment'. More recently, Oleribe et al. (2018) have highlighted how the WHO definition is also hard to measure.

With reference to older people living with and managing chronic disease, Fallon and Karlawish (2019) argue that the WHO's definition is not inclusive enough since it does not account for this part of the life course, and that it thus needs to be revised and updated. The world has changed a lot since the definition was first enshrined in the WHO constitution in 1948. At that point average global life expectancy was about 48 years for men and 53 for women (Fallon and Karlawish, 2019). People in many countries now live a lot longer than this: as of 2022, global life expectancy was nearly 70 years for men and just over 74 for women (World Bank, 2023). Fallon and Karlawish (2019: npn) argue that 'having disease and feeling healthy are no longer mutually exclusive, especially for older adults' (although by no means exclusively), such that many older adults are likely to describe themselves as being healthy despite living with chronic disease.

Philosopher Catherine McDonald (2023) points to the problematic use of the notion of completeness in the WHO's definition. She argues that this is probably the biggest problem with it in that completeness is very difficult to identify and measure, is not a universal concept, and can be understood in different ways. McDonald (2023: npn) also points out that 'while the inclusion of total well-being under the WHO definition of health is one of its attractions, it is also its greatest weakness. By including subjective well-being into the concept of health, the concept ultimately dissolves into a myriad personal subjectivities among which there is no obvious priority.' She concludes that, 'by attempting to include all aspects of life impinging on human well-being into the concept of health, the WHO definition ultimately becomes unintelligible'. Some would view this as a rather harsh critique; but McDonald has a point and similar observations have been made by others.

Despite calls to do so, the WHO has not yet revised its definition of health. Recently, however, others have attempted to do so. Writing in the *Pan African Medical Journal*, Oleribe et al. (2018: 3) suggest that health be defined as 'a satisfactory and acceptable state of physical (biological), mental (intellectual), emotional (psychological), economic (financial), and social (societal) well-being'. They describe this as an all-encompassing definition, yet it does not include several aspects or dimensions of health that some people think are important; for example, spiritual and environmental health. However, they do go on to say that health is 'the state of having the overall physical, mental, emotional, and social ability to add value not just to one's self, but to society, resulting in the development of a better and sustainable world where things work, people live in harmony and community existence is enhanced' (2018: 3). This, too, might be criticized for being idealistic.

Health as a social construct

We have already noted in this chapter that health can be viewed as a social construct, and this is the perspective which generally dominates the discussion in this book.

Understanding health as socially constructed is an important consideration for definitions of health and for trying to understand what health is about. Social constructionist perspectives on health allow for subjectivity and reject the existence of an external 'truth' about what health is. From a social construction perspective, health is what people believe it to be and is defined by how people act and understand it. Viewing health in this way enables us to take into account the various different ways that people conceive of health and also to understand it as a fluid, organic concept (Warwick-Booth et al., 2021).

Socialization processes contribute to, and influence, our ideas about health. As Wills (2023) observes, different views about what health is can co-exist within a single society, dependent on how ideas are passed down over time, and are influenced by things like culture and tradition. Understanding health as a social construct therefore allows us to consider the manifold ways that health can be understood and experienced. It also allows for consideration of the various factors that affect and influence health. As Warwick-Booth et al. (2021: 16) argue, 'from a social constructionist perspective the meaning of health is created (constructed) through the way that we, as social beings, interact and the language that we use'. From a social constructionist perspective, understandings of health are created and evolve through discourse, and it is possible for many different understandings of health to co-exist even whilst they might, at times, seem to be at odds with each other.

One way of appreciating health as a social construct is to look at how ideas about health have changed over time. Tapper (2021) describes changing understandings of health in the West from prehistoric times (see Table 1.1 for further information).

Table 1.1 charts changes in understandings about health in the West from before the time of the written word to around 200 years ago. Since then, understandings of health in many places in the world have been dominated by scientific perspectives such as, initially, the biomedical model of health and, latterly, the biopsychosocial model of health (Tapper, 2021). Both of these perspectives will be discussed in more detail in Chapter 3.

Table 1.1: Changing understandings of health in the West over time

Time period	Examples of understandings about health
Prehistoric (prior to around 3000 years BC)	Archaeological evidence from prehistoric skulls reveals the practice of making holes in them, which is presumed to have been done to alleviate physical or psychological symptoms. It is believed that the practice, known as *trepanation*, may also have resulted from a ritual linked to spiritual beliefs.
Ancient history (from around 3000 years BC to around 500 AD)	Ancient civilizations acquired a lot of understanding about the causes and treatment of disease, although this was often thought to involve supernatural influences. In some parts of the world, ill health began to be understood as an imbalance of certain things within the body, which then needed rebalancing to achieve health (as in Ayurvedic medicine and traditional Chinese medicine). The understanding of the ancient Greeks moved from a belief in prayer and sacrifice as a means for healing to the Hippocratic belief that ill health had natural rather than supernatural causes. This transition is viewed as the foundation of modern 'western' medicine. Another popular practice of the time was bloodletting, advocated by Galen, who believed that drawing blood would restore the balance between the four humours (the bodily fluids of phlegm, black bile, yellow bile and blood) and thereby restore health.
The Middle Ages (around 500 AD to around 1500 AD)	During this period the ideas of Hippocrates and Galen continued to be influential, with bloodletting remaining popular. Alongside this, supernatural ideas persisted, in witchcraft, astrology and the belief in a higher power causing disease as punishment. The advance of Christianity led to a belief in prayer for healing, care of the sick as a duty of the church, and the first iterations of modern hospitals.
Early Modern (or Renaissance) period (around 1300 AD to around 1600 AD)	This relatively short period brought a lot of changes in understandings about health. There was a resurgence of ancient Greek philosophy, literature and art alongside major advances in the arts and science, in particular the experimental method. The first human dissection took place during this time, becoming routine practice in Europe by the mid-1550s. Ideas of the mind and body as separate entities (derived from the French philosopher René Descartes and referred to as 'dualism') began to dominate.
Late Modern period (from around the 1800s)	Understandings of the origins of disease advanced further, with miasma theory (in which ill health is caused by breathing 'bad air') being gradually replaced by germ theory (in which ill health is caused by organisms such as bacteria).

Source: Adapted from Tapper (2021: 5–7)

As we can see, the way that health is viewed and experienced in the social world changes over time, with implications for the ways in which health is understood. Table 1.1 chiefly focuses on the western history of health, but health is a universal concept and understandings of it vary considerably both within and between societies. Social construction takes into account people's so-called 'health cultures' (behaviours, traditions, customs, shared experiences, etc.) (Nanjunda, 2015: 175). Different understandings are apparent in the way that health is supported or maintained in different contexts, but when health is considered more broadly, different ways of promoting and improving it come into play. Nevertheless, as sociologist Sigrun Olafsdottir (2013) notes, although social constructionism insists that ideas about health are constantly (re)constructed through our social interactions, there is an 'objective' element to this given that our health also has a biological (or physiological) component to it. After all, we experience many aspects of health as corporeal beings.

Health as a moral phenomenon

The pursuit of health has long been associated with ideas about being good, virtuous and responsible (Crossley, 2003; Lupton and Peterson, 1996), and morality has been a significant aspect of the social understandings of health referred to in the previous section. The idea that people have a moral and personal responsibility to maintain their health is echoed in the neoliberal policy that underpins many aspects of health promotion and provision today, particularly in more wealthy countries. Weight is an area where this is very apparent. For example, contemporary discourse around obesity tends to focus on individuals and personal responsibility, reflecting moral assumptions about what people should (or should not) eat and do (or do not) eat (Ristovski-Slijepcevic et al., 2010). Lifestyle choices become labelled as 'good' or 'bad', reflecting underlying moral beliefs about what is right or wrong which are in turn informed by socio-cultural norms (Frederick et al., 2016). Fatness brings more moral judgements and stigma associated with ideas about laziness and greed, themselves informed by ancient ideas about sin (sloth, gluttony) (Wathne, 2014; Pausé, 2018). If people do not behave in what are defined as 'healthy' ways they risk being blamed and discriminated against. We become morally obligated to do everything we can to stay healthy (Brady et al., 2013). A good citizen is therefore someone who looks after their health to the best of their ability and who avoids putting demands on healthcare services.

The pursuit of health is framed as an imperative and as something which is in the control of the individual (Lupton and Peterson, 1996). Robert Crawford (2006: 402) refers to this as 'healthism', arguing that being healthy is 'understood as an intricate and demanding project' which requires self-discipline, self-monitoring and self-management of certain behaviours (Welsh, 2011). These ideas perpetuate personal responsibility for health and are rooted in an ideology of individualism (Wilkinson, 2006), resulting in the health-conscious subject (Ayo, 2012). The discourse of citizenship constructs the good citizen as a healthy citizen (Peterson et al., 2010) and emphasizes maintaining good individual health as a civic duty (Gustafson, 2011; Green et al., 2012). People who do not fit with this are constructed as deviant, a drain on resources and a burden to society when they experience ill health and need treatment or support. All of this works to draw attention away from the social and structural determinants of health which we will consider in more detail in Chapter 4.

The moralization of health is evident in mass media as well as professional discourse (Arnoldi, 2009), such that the pursuit of health becomes the pursuit of morality (Roy, 2008). These neoliberal ideas are notably more prevalent in 'westernized' countries; however, epidemiological transition (where, as people become wealthier and live longer, chronic diseases cause more death than infectious diseases [Mackenbach, 2022]) is resulting in the pervasion of these ideas in the global south too, as the incidence and prevalence of non-communicable diseases such as cancers and cardiovascular disease increase, particularly among the emergent middle classes. Of course, this largely promotes the notion of health as existing solely within a physical dimension – our bodies.

Lay perspectives and lived experience

We have already alluded to the importance of lay perspectives, and in this final section of the chapter we will consider them in more depth. Lay perspectives on health are an important feature of health as a social construct and a key component in the social model of health (see Chapter 3). Lay perspectives can help us to further appreciate the complexities of health and health experience. Also described as 'lay knowledge' (Earle, 2007), 'lay expertise' (Martin, 2008), 'lay concepts' or 'lay beliefs', they can be distinguished from professional or theoretical ideas about health. Here we will use 'lay perspectives' as a generic term for the purposes of discussion.

Lay perspectives on health are influenced by many factors such as experience, culture, age, gender, geographical location, levels of education, socioeconomic position, mass media and so on. All of these can, and do, influence how people think and feel about health, and how they experience it (Manstead, 2018). Social media has also had an increasing influence on ideas about health over the past couple of decades (Baker and Rojeck, 2019), as seen in the promotion of a singular idealized image of what a healthy (perfect) body should look like (i.e. for men – muscular, toned, low in body fat) (Hilkens et al., 2021). Before reading further, please take some time to do Pause for Reflection 1.2.

Pause for Reflection 1.2

Take some time out to think about different people you know or have met. How do/might their personal ideas about health differ or cohere? You could, for example, compare an older person with a child or a teenager. Think about the different people in your neighbourhood or workplace. What factors might influence their perspectives on health? What about someone living in relative poverty compared to someone who is wealthy? Also, reflect on your own ideas about health. How have they changed over time? What factors have influenced that change?

A significant amount of recent research has been done on lay perspectives; however, there is some seminal work that is worth consideration here. In Chapter 2, we will look more closely at Mildred Blaxter's work from the early 1990s on lay concepts of health, but around the same time social psychologist Wendy Stainton-Rogers (1991) carried out research into lay understandings of health and illness and, as a result, offered seven different accounts of health as follows:

- *Body as machine* (links with medical understandings of health viewing the body as something that can break down and need fixing, or that needs maintenance)
- *Body under siege* (external factors influencing health, e.g. germs, viewing the body as something that needs protecting from negative outside forces)
- *Inequality of access* (for example, lack of access to medical or healthcare services; ill health is viewed as a product of social injustice)
- *Cultural critique* (linked with ideas about exploitation and oppression; health is explained in terms of power, status and wealth; 'poor health is the product of inequality, exploitation and disadvantage' (Stainton-Rogers 1991: 139)
- *Health promotion* (focused more on health than illness; concerned with lifestyle but also linked with ideas about collective responsibility for health)
- *Robust individualism* (linked with rights to a satisfying life and ideas about individual freedom)
- *Willpower* (linked with ideas about individual control, viewing health in terms of individual responsibility and maintaining a positive mindset)

About twenty years later, health psychologists Felicity Bishop and Lucy Yardley (2010: 272) identified three major themes across different studies of lay definitions of health: health as the absence of disease ('health is something that one *is*'); health as the ability to perform daily activities ('health is something that one *has*'); and health as the experience of vitality and balance ('health can be something that one *does*'). More recently, Svalastog et al. (2017) identified three qualities of health that characterize lay perspectives:

wholeness, pragmatism and individualism, further described in Table 1.2.

As can be seen from the research findings presented so far, it is not atypical for lay perspectives to subsume and reproduce medicalized and scientific ideas about what health is (Woodall and Cross, 2022). However, they often also reflect other ideas about the factors influencing health, for example incorporating beliefs about evil spirits, curses and witchcraft (Moorley et al., 2016; Tedeschi, 2017). Chinese culture promotes the idea of balance between yin and yang, whilst traditional Indian healing systems refer to the idea of karma (Gopalkrishnan, 2018).

Our history (individual and collective) also impacts on our ideas about health. A South African study exploring young people's perspectives on health found that ideas of personal freedom were important; indeed, the researchers chose a quote from one participant as the title for their article: 'To be healthy to me is to be free.' This is perhaps not surprising given that, prior to 1994, South Africa restricted the majority of the population's rights and freedoms under the strict policy

Table 1.2: Svalastog et al.'s (2017) lay perspectives on health

Quality	Explanation
Wholeness	Health is viewed in a holistic way as inherent to all aspects of life, including family, work and community. It is seen as a resource for living and as the ability to function. Being able to live according to one's personal values is also regarded as important.
Pragmatism	Health is viewed as a relative experience, as what people might reasonably expect in the light of their personal situations (age, health conditions, social circumstances). Other positive values in life can compensate for disability or disease.
Individualism	Health is seen as a very personal phenomenon dependent on who you are as an individual. But feeling close to other people and feeling part of a community or society is an important element of this.

Source: Adapted from Svalastog et al. (2017: 434)

of apartheid that treated Blacks as second-class citizens (De Jong et al., 2019).

With reference to Indigenous health, Dykhuizen et al. (2022) highlight how the legacy of colonialization has influenced the contemporary health experiences of First Nations people in Canada. The authors highlight the importance of the concept of intersectionality for gaining a better understanding of how to meet the health needs of Indigenous people. Theories of intersectionality argue that we all have different identities bound up in aspects of who we are (for example, gender, race and sexuality), and that such 'markers of difference intersect and reflect social structures of oppression and privilege such as sexism, racism and heteronormativity' (Kelly et al., 2021: 187).

A final concept to note here is that of 'healthworlds', which relates to how people think about, experience and behave in relation to their own health. An individual's healthworld is influenced by our shared social healthworlds (Germond and Cochrane, 2010). Healthworlds are organic; they evolve and change as people, communities and societies change. Therefore, as Adams et al. (2019) note, multiple healthworlds can co-exist within one society. Germond and Cochrane (2010: 316) argue that the notion of healthworlds 'requires that we be attentive to the complex whole of human well-being'.

To take one example, Nadal et al. (2022) explored the concepts of healthworlds in relation to understandings of rabies in India. Alongside some appreciation of rabies as a biological infection, there were strong beliefs that human rabies is a social illness caused by the goddess Hadkai Mata, who infects dogs with rabies and makes them bite people who misbehave. The authors argue that these beliefs are 'deeply embedded in local social, cultural and religious settings' (Nadal et al., 2022: 1). Similarly, research in the United States exploring racial and ethnic differences in attitudes towards prescription medication has shown how minority groups have healthworlds in which confidence in the efficacy of such medication is low, with many expressing a preference for alternative solutions, as compared with white counterparts in the same study. Notions of connectedness – with each other and the natural world – are central to the worldviews of Indigenous communities in the US and Canada (Walls et al., 2022). These cases illustrate the fact that health-worlds are various, differing and context-dependent, and reinforce the importance of decolonizing ideas about health and taking lay perspectives into account (Dykhuizen et al., 2022).

It should now be apparent that, as Green et al. (2019) argue, lay perspectives on health are sophisticated and complex, going far beyond ideas about health as simply the absence of disease and infirmity. The result is a rich variety of views on health that need to be taken into account (Cross et al., 2021a). We will, then, necessarily return to lay perspectives throughout the book, as they are interwoven in the various discussions and debates about what health is.

Case Study 1: Young women, risk and health (Cross, 2013)

Young women's risky health practices (smoking, alcohol misuse, risky sexual behaviour, etc.) are generally viewed as problematic. Research carried out in the north of England exploring young women's (aged 18–24 years) ideas about health and risk found that they attributed different meanings to their so-called 'risky' health behaviours. Although their perspectives reflected common themes relating to health, such as moralism, healthy citizenship and health as a feminine pursuit, they also conceptualized their 'unhealthy' practices in alternative ways – as resistant to societal expectations, as expressions of freedom and agency, and as bringing meaning to their lived experiences. This illustrates the importance of understanding lay perspectives on health in relation to supporting the promotion of young women's health. Their experiences and perspectives need to be taken in account in the risk communication strategies and health promotion interventions aimed at them.

Summary

This chapter has considered the concept of health and introduced some key ideas that will recur throughout the rest of the book. We have started to explore the notion of health as complex and contested, acknowledging that we cannot propose a one-size-fits-all approach to defining health given that it is situated within personal experiences and sociocultural contexts, and therefore means different things to different people. This chapter has highlighted the socially constructed nature of health, which will be a key theme in the subsequent discussions. It has also emphasized the central role that lay perspectives have in any exploration of what health is. Appreciating different concepts of health is important for those who work in the health field, and beyond. It enables us to better understand how to promote, support and improve health for everyone, including ourselves. The next chapter will consider different dimensions of health.

Further reading

Chapter 1: Health and Health Promotion. In Cross, R. and Woodall, J. (2024) *Green and Tones's Health Promotion: Planning and Strategies.* 5th edition. London, Sage, pp. 8–59.

This comprehensive chapter considers the question of what health is within the context of promoting health, and explores related issues such as equity, power, empowerment and ethics in significant depth.

2
Dimensions of Health

Introduction

As discussed in Chapter 1, health can be thought of in various ways. One common way is to think of it as existing within different dimensions, each of which focuses on a different aspect of health. There are several frameworks on dimensions of health in the wider literature. You might come across five-dimensional frameworks which typically include the physical, spiritual, emotional, social and mental dimensions of health. In a discussion of what constitutes wellness, however, Deborah Stoewen (2017: 861) refers to eight dimensions – physical, intellectual, emotional, social, spiritual, vocational, financial, and environmental – all of which she describes as being 'mutually interdependent'.

In this chapter several different dimensions of health will be considered, each in turn. At the outset it is acknowledged that this is a highly theoretical, conceptual approach to take since each dimension is not entirely discrete and because different dimensions of health will overlap, intersect and interact to some extent. Nevertheless, the following dimensions of health will be considered – physical health, mental health, spiritual health, emotional health, social health and societal health. Finally, the notion of holistic health will be outlined and discussed as a means of bringing the different dimensions together as well as offering a new perspective on health which considers the 'whole person'. Lay perspectives on health will be intertwined throughout the discussion drawing on research and evidence from around the world and taking into account the multitude of factors that impact on ideas about health (for example, culture, age and gender).

Physical health

As we saw in the previous chapter, physical health can often take precedence when we try to conceptualize health. This is for several reasons, which will be explored at various points in the book. For many people health is about being able to function and so it is conceived as having to do with the condition of our physical bodies (Hjelm, 2010) – whether we feel well and able enough to do what we want and need to do. At least that has been the focus historically, particularly over the past couple of centuries in so-called 'western' countries. This is because, as noted by Woodall and Cross (2022), we live in physical bodies that get ill, become unfit and incur injuries. As Jane Wills (2023) explains, physical health is about not being ill, about being fit – essentially it is about the absence of disease, injury or disability. Physical health is important for survival and becomes more of a priority in situations where it is harder to maintain but crucial for existence (think of resource-poor environments where people are simply trying to survive from day to day, or living in relative poverty, disadvantage and deprivation).

As Scriven (2017: 8) suggests, physical health is 'perhaps the most obvious dimension of health and is concerned with the mechanistic functioning of the body'. As discussed in Chapter 1, many lay perspectives refer to health in the physical dimension – as about being able to function, work, play, etc. Blaxter's (2010) seminal research on British lay concepts of health in the 1980s identified several themes relating to physical health, including: not being ill (not experiencing symptoms or having to visit the doctor), being physically fit, being able to function, having energy and vitality and having the ability to recover quickly from being unwell or injured. In addition, health was directly linked to lifestyle or behaviour, so being healthy meant looking after your own health, for example by eating a healthy diet or being physically active.

Locating health in the purely physical realm leads to a focus on illness, disease and disability and to an assumption that if physical health is lacking then health cannot exist. A concern with physical health is the primary focus of a lot of medical and healthcare services, which centre on making people physically well again or treating accidents and injury. Nevertheless, a person may have a disability, be injured or diagnosed with an illness and still say that they are healthy (Warwick-Booth et al., 2021). Conversely, a person might be physically robust yet report poor health due to mental distress. Another theme from Blaxter's work on lay perspectives was health despite disease, where health is considered to exist when people are able to 'successfully cope with a chronic condition such as diabetes or arthritis' (Tapper, 2021: 3).

Physical health (or the lack of it) is frequently used as a measure of health largely at the expense of other dimensions of health. It is very easy to access huge amounts of information about the physical health of people at local, regional and global levels, which enables comparisons to be made between and within countries. The Global Burden of Disease (GBD) is an example of the foregrounding of the dimension of physical health. First set up over thirty years ago, the GBD is a study that assesses disease, injuries and risk factors in more than 200 countries around the world (Murray, 2022). Measures such as this allow for comparisons to be made between countries based on physical health outcomes reflected primarily by mortality (death) and morbidity (disease, injury and risk factors) rates. The GBD is used to quantify health loss, largely through a focus on corporeal experience or physical health outcomes in relation to disability, illness and injury. This then informs the enhancement of national and global health systems and attempts to reduce global disparities in health outcomes (GBD, 2023).

At the time of writing this chapter, the most recent GBD data available was from 2019 (because the global COVID-19 pandemic had delayed the process of gathering and reporting data). The 2019 data was reported from 204 countries and territories on 369 diseases and injuries and eighty-seven risk factors (The Lancet, 2023). The results showed that, in general, the health of the world's population was 'steadily improving', as measured by global life expectancy (up from 67.2 years in 2000 to 73.5 years in 2019), the increase of 'healthy life expectancy in 202 of 204 countries and territories', and the increase 'in 21 countries [of] healthy life expectancy at birth ... by more than 10 years between 1990 and 2019, with gains of up to 19.1 years' (The Lancet, 2020: 1129). This, and other data like it, illustrates the continued importance of the physical dimension of health due to it being relatively easy to measure, directly compare and track. However, such data seldom takes into account the multi-dimensional nature of health.

Mental health

Mental health has been receiving more and more interest in recent years, driven by several factors, including celebrity attention, media campaigns and a greater appreciation of the importance of this dimension of health. Alongside this increase in awareness we have witnessed an increase in mental ill health. Mental health is not easy to define, considerably less so compared with physical health (Cross and Woodall, 2024). It is, however, increasingly salient in terms of health experience and outcomes. At the simplest level mental health is concerned with how we feel and what, and how, we think. Mental health is therefore related to emotional health. It also has to do with how we cope with stress, how resilient we are and the extent to which we can be active, productive members of our community/society. All these ideas are picked up in the World Health Organization's definition of mental health (Box 2.1).

Box 2.1: World Health Organization (2014: npn) definition of mental health

'A state of well-being in which every individual realizes [their] own potential, can cope with the normal stresses of life, can work productively and fruitfully, and is able to make a contribution to [their] community.'

Scriven (2017: 8) defines mental health as 'the ability to think clearly and coherently', whilst for Wills (2023: 3) 'mental health refers to a positive sense of purpose and an underlying belief in one's one worth, for example, feeling good, feeling able to cope'. For some, then, mental health is solely concerned with our cognitive ability; for others it is also about how we feel. Mental health is therefore closely related to emotional and social health, although we can usefully consider it as a separate and distinct dimension of health for the purposes of this discussion.

Many people, such as Prince et al. (2007), argue that there is no health without mental health. The links between physical health and mental health are evident. When we are physically unwell or experience any kind of physical trauma it has an impact on how we feel. In addition, when we feel down, depressed or stressed this often leads to physical (somatic) symptoms. The COVID-19 pandemic was detrimental to mental health in many ways. A literature review reported by Hossain et al. (2020) showed that people who had been affected by COVID-19 experienced a high burden of mental health issues, including increased depression and anxiety. Boredom, fear and panic were also mental manifestations of distress, particularly during the early stages of the pandemic; then came the devastating effects of loss of livelihoods, bereavements and increases in domestic violence, as described by researchers from India (Kumar and Nayar, 2020) but certainly not peculiar to that country. The mental health of healthcare workers was also negatively impacted, with research showing that they experienced trauma and worse mental health than the general public and had an increased susceptibility to psychological problems at a global level (Vizheh et al., 2020).

Blaxter's (2010) research findings have implications in relation to the concept of health as energy and vitality, which are important features of positive mental health. This is not just a physical idea rooted in fitness – it is also concerned with feeling alert and having an enthusiasm for life, both of which are linked to mental health experience. Another lay perspective in Blaxter's findings concerned health as psychosocial well-being, which is specific to having good mental health and feeling happy or relaxed. Mental health is about the mind, but the mind is inextricably linked to physical health. Consider, for example, the placebo and nocebo effects (see Box 2.2). Placebo effects are beneficial whilst nocebo effects tend to be harmful (Planès et al., 2016). Research shows that placebo treatments can reduce the side effects of cancer therapies and even the symptoms of cancer itself (such as fatigue, nausea and pain); they can also reduce the perception of severity of asthma symptoms (Kaptchuk and Miller, 2015). Another example of the strong link between the dimensions of mental health and physical health is 'somatization', where mental health problems manifest as physical ailments (O'Sullivan, 2015). Physical signs of emotional or mental distress are described as 'somatic'; for example, someone might present with pain or other physical symptoms that are actually caused by anxiety or stress.

Mental disorders* are a significant burden on global health, impacting on the general welfare of societies across the world. As of 2019 it was estimated that the burden of mental

---

* 'Mental disorders' is the term used by the Global Burden of Disease; however, it is acknowledged that people can, and do, live positively with mental ill health and that such language can be stigmatizing and discriminatory. The challenges of mental health are exacerbated by structural issues such as poverty, lack of (meaningful) employment and lack of access to appropriate support.

> **Box 2.2: Placebo and nocebo effects (from Tapper, 2021)**
>
> *Placebo effect* – 'a beneficial effect bought about by a substance or treatment which cannot be attributed to the properties of that substance or treatment and is therefore thought to occur due to the person's belief in the substance or treatment' (p. 8)
>
> *Nocebo effect* – 'a harmful effect brought about by a substance or treatment which cannot be attributed to the physical properties of that substance or treatment and is therefore attributed to the person's belief in the substance or treatment' (p. 9)

health as measured by disability-adjusted years (DALYs) had more than tripled compared to previous estimates (Arias et al., 2022). This was before the inevitable impact of the COVID-19 pandemic on mental health. Given that mental health is a key component of the health experience and, as Arias et al. (2022) argue, essential for people to flourish, clearly it is a significant dimension of health. As will be discussed in Chapter 4, mental health is affected by many different factors, and good mental health may be undermined by insecurity of any kind, for example economic, political or social.

Spiritual health

Spiritual health is another dimension of health that has been receiving more attention in academic circles in recent years. It is closely connected to mental health and emotional health as it is related to how we make sense of, and find purpose in, life. The idea of purpose is picked up by Wills (2023: 3), who states that 'spiritual health is the recognition and ability to put into practice moral or religious principles or beliefs, and the feeling of having a "higher" purpose in life'. In cases where spiritually like-minded people meet together, spiritual health may also be linked with social health.

There is an absence of an agreed definition of spiritual health despite the recognition of its importance (Jaberi et al., 2017), but, as Cross and Woodall (2024: 15) point out, 'many people have asserted that any serious consideration of positive health must include the spiritual dimension'. Spiritual health is concerned with cognition (how and what we think) and affect (how we feel) but it is also linked to faith and beliefs which are frequently, but by no means always, manifest in religious or faith practices. Fisher et al. (2000) stated that there are four domains of spiritual health – one concerned with the self, one with community, one with the environment and one with a higher power; whilst Scriven (2017: 8) observes that, 'for some people, spiritual health might be connected with religious beliefs and practices; for other people, it might be associated with personal creeds, principles of behaviour and ways of achieving peace of mind and being at peace with oneself'. Such a definition covers many different things.

In a study exploring experts' ideas about spiritual health in Iran (Ghaderi et al., 2018), the participants distinguished between spirituality and spiritual health, characterizing the latter as follows:

- Affecting physical, mental and social health
- Dominating other aspects of health
- Having religious and existential approaches
- Being perceptible in how people behave
- As being able to be enhanced and improved

While the five characteristics of spirituality were considered to be:

- Meaning
- Value
- Transcendence (existence beyond the physical)
- Connecting (with oneself, others, the environment, God/a supreme power)
- Becoming (growth and progress in life)

Interestingly, in this study, most of the participants recognized human connection with God as the most important part of the definition of spiritual health (Ghaderi et al., 2018). Indeed, in some cultures especially (Iran being an example), spiritual health is considered to be a major component of people's subjective health status and experience (Farshadnia et al., 2018). The findings are, of course, likely to be culturally and context specific, which points to the subjective nature of health in all of its dimensions.

Research indicates that spiritual health can have a positive impact on risk-taking in young people and that it provides protective benefits. For example, in a study by Hatala et al. (2021) involving adolescents in Saskatchewan, Canada, spiritual health seemed to mitigate against a range of health-risk behaviours such as smoking, drug and alcohol use and early sexual intercourse. These findings are consistent with research in other contexts. A study in the Czech Republic found the same in relation to adolescent smoking and alcohol consumption, but also that religious attendance (defined by how often a participant attended church or religious sessions) played an important part in mitigating against risk behaviours (Malinakova et al., 2018).

Despite the importance of the spiritual dimension of health, it has often been neglected in the training of healthcare professionals. Bhatt (2020) concluded that simplifying the definitions of spirituality and spiritual health could enable smoother discussions about this dimension in the training of the healthcare workforce in India, with a resultant effect on the ease of discussion about spirituality and spiritual health in communities with diverse faiths and beliefs. Similarly, researchers in Australia have noted that the spiritual dimension of health has been 'neglected in policy and practice' (Love et al., 2017: 179). Drawing on research using Indigenous and non-Indigenous methodologies, Love et al. found that the Indigenous perspective 'proposed that spiritual well-being is founded in The Dreaming, informs everyday relationships and can impact on health'. On the other hand, the non-Indigenous perspective 'suggested that spiritual well-being is shaped by culture and religion, is of increased importance as one ages, and can improve coping and resilience stressors' (Love et al., 2017: 179).

Unlike in more secular cultures, spirituality is at the core of Aboriginal (Indigenous) identity; everything is viewed as being (inter)connected. The Dreaming refers to sacred stories passed down from generation to generation that talk about the interconnectedness of all things (people, nature, celestial bodies, etc.) and give meaning to life (Love et al., 2017). The spiritual dimension of health is also reflected in beliefs about the malevolence of the 'evil eye', which appear in many cultures across the world (Alqarni, 2020).

Emotional health

Emotional health is strongly associated with mental health. It is concerned with feelings and affect. Whilst mental health can be viewed as being about cognition, or our ability to think and use our brains effectively, emotional health is often conceived of as being about feelings and mood or our emotional state. Scriven (2017: 8) defines emotional health as 'the ability to recognize emotions such as fear, joy, grief and anger, and to express such emotions appropriately', adding that 'emotional (or affective) health also means coping with stress, tension, depression and anxiety'. So emotional health is about the ability to recognize, express and manage our emotions, and to be able to cope with what life throws at us. The link to mental health is clear again here with regards to coping. Wills (2023) goes a little further in her definition of emotional health. Whilst recognizing that it is concerned with 'the ability to feel, recognize and give voice to feelings', Wills (2023: 3) goes on to say that emotional health is about being able to 'develop and sustain relationships, for example, being loved'. In this sense then, emotional health is also strongly connected to social health.

Blaxter's (2010) work on lay perspectives implied that emotional health is important to people. Whilst emotional health was not explicitly identified as a key theme, feeling happy was highlighted under the theme of 'psychosocial well-being' as being key to health. Other research has shown the importance of this dimension in people's ideas about health. For example, US college students identified the absence of stress and anxiety as a major contributory factor in their understandings of health (Downey and Chang, 2013). Both stress and anxiety, whilst associated with mental health, can be emotional states or feelings: people will say they are 'feeling stressed' or anxious. The COVID-19 pandemic increased anxiety, not just for those who were infected and became sick, but also for the general population (Magnúsdóttir et al., 2022). This phenomenon was seen in many different countries and contexts.

Emotional health is also about how we feel about ourselves, or our self-esteem. Social media, whilst having many positive effects, has also been shown to increase anxiety around many different things, such as body image (Lenza, 2020). Canadian authors Tremblay et al. (2021) concur with this in their discussion of how interacting with social media platforms such as Snapchat increases feelings of body dissatisfaction for many adolescents. Research in India has shown how taking selfies increases social anxiety, decreases self-confidence and leads to a decrease in feelings of being physically attractive, particularly for women (Shome et al., 2020).

Emotional health is often connected with feelings of well-being (Forgeard et al., 2011) and happiness, emotional experiences that inform personal perspectives about health. Chapters 5 and 6 discuss both of these related concepts in much more depth.

Emotional resilience, sometimes referred to as psychological resilience (Bozdağ and Ergün, 2021), is also a feature of emotional health. Whilst resilience is a complex idea and open to being contested, it is generally considered to be important for recovering from adversity. It has been described as the ability to 'bounce back' from negative emotions or events (Yang et al., 2022), or 'the capability to quickly adjust negative emotions and successfully overcome a difficult situation' (Wang et al., 2021: 3). This returns us to the idea of coping. For example, Tranter et al.'s (2021) research shows how emotional resilience can help when dealing with adverse childhood experiences or post-traumatic stress. It is about being able to adapt and deal with stressful and upsetting situations and events, whether past or present. Emotional resilience was also found to be an important factor in how healthcare workers experienced, and responded to, the global COVID-19 pandemic.

Research in Turkey has highlighted the direct causal links between emotional resilience and other dimensions of health, such as the physical and mental. For example, emotional resilience was found to improve when physical health needs such as sufficient sleep were met (Bozdağ and Ergűn, 2021). In addition, positive emotions and life satisfaction, associated with good mental health, were also found to be important factors – when these were improved, resilience levels were higher. As mentioned at the start of this chapter, the dimensions of health overlap and interact and should not be considered as acting in isolation.

Social health

The social dimension of health is concerned with the relationships and connections we have with other people in our communities and with the health of society as a whole. It may not be surprising by now to learn that social health is complex and not easy to define; however, as Cross and Woodall (2024) argue, it is integral to experiences of health. Social health has two key components: the social health of the individual and the social health of society (Warwick-Booth et al., 2021). The social health of society will be specifically discussed in the next section, on societal health; here we focus on the social health of the individual.

Alongside the other key themes in her work on lay perspectives, Blaxter (2010) found that health was also conceived in terms of social relationships – as having good relationships with other people and being able to experience reciprocity. In Svalastog et al.'s (2017) conceptualization of lay perspectives, feeling close to other people and being part of a community or society was an important factor for health. In a Nepalese study focusing on women, Yang et al. (2018) found that concepts of health were related to peace in the family, i.e. the absence of disruption and discord, which again highlights the importance of relationships in social health. For Scriven (2017: 8) social health is about the 'ability to make and maintain relationships with other people', but it is also about having people to talk to and do things with, as well as having a sense of being supported by others such as friends and family (Wills, 2023).

The social health of an individual can therefore be said to be suffering if they feel isolated and have no one to depend on, or if they lack meaningful connections with other people. Research shows that loneliness is a significant risk factor in relation to the likelihood of dying earlier than would otherwise be expected. Loneliness, understood as 'the subjective feeling of being alone (perceived isolation)' (Perissinotto et al., 2019: 657), has been identified as a major public health issue because it is also associated with an increased risk for depression, high blood pressure, cardiovascular disease and stroke (Lederman, 2023). Loneliness is not exclusive to older people, but the risk of experiencing it does increase as we age. In a Dutch study on excess mortality in older adults, Holwerda et al. (2016) found that loneliness and depression were associated with a greater likelihood of dying earlier than expected, particularly among older men.

On the other hand, having access to social support and social connection leads to better health outcomes. For example, in a study by Freak-Poli et al. (2022), women who were not isolated and who had high levels of social support reported higher health-related quality of life compared to those who were isolated, had low levels of social support and were lonely. Many things can mitigate feelings of social isolation and provide social support in times of crises; for example, a Spanish study has demonstrated the importance of social media use in this regard (Rosen et al., 2022). Social media can enable meaningful connections with other people, promoting social support and providing opportunities to form new friendships.

Social support and connection are features of 'social capital', which is a consistent predictor of better health (Wind and Villalonga-Olives, 2018). There are various definitions of social capital in the wider literature, but it is generally understood to be about the connections between people, trust in others, reciprocity, community cohesion and civic engagement (Ehsan et al., 2019), all of which are pertinent to individual social health. A useful way of understanding social capital is to draw a distinction between structural social capital and cognitive social capital. Structural social capital is about networks in society and the quality of relationships within those networks, whilst cognitive social capital is about a person's 'perception of the level of interpersonal trust within a group and reciprocal norms' (Yuan et al., 2021: 501).

The social restrictions that were put in place in many countries during the early months of the COVID-19 pandemic had a detrimental impact on the social health of many people, leading to increased feelings of isolation and the loss of social support networks (Millman et al., 2020). In many ways the global pandemic had a detrimental impact on social capital due to the enforced social distancing and isolation. In other ways the pandemic had a positive impact on social capital resulting in beneficial outcomes, such as connecting with other people in virtual environments and an increase in volunteerism. In addition, social capital acted as a protective buffer for some. For example, in the United States, higher levels of social capital seemed to be associated with a lower spread of the virus (and subsequently lower cases of infection) thanks to community engagement in social distancing and personal hygiene practices, which arguably resulted from a greater concern for the welfare of other people – a feature of communities characterized by high levels of trust and better relationships (Makridis and Wu, 2021).

Societal health

The dimension of social health is essentially about what it means to be a healthy society. While there are different conceptualizations about what constitutes a healthy society, there is general agreement that it will be one in which the needs of the worst off are prioritized (Felton, 2021), in which there is greater equality, and in which everyone can flourish to the best of their potential (including in terms of health) (Horton, 2016). Wills (2023: 3) states that 'societal health refers to the link between health and the way a society is structured. This includes the basic infrastructure necessary for health (such as shelter, peace, food, income) and the degree of integration or division within society.' Box 2.3 offers a more detailed explanation of societal health.

Box 2.3: Societal health (Scriven, 2017: 8)

'[A] person's health is inextricably related to everything surrounding that person. It is impossible to be healthy in a sick society that does not provide the resources for basic physical and emotional needs. For example, people obviously cannot be healthy if they cannot afford necessities like food, clothing and shelter, but neither can they be healthy in countries of extreme political oppression where basic human rights are denied. Women cannot be healthy when their contribution to society is undervalued, and neither black nor white can be healthy in a racist society where racism undermines human worth, self-esteem and social relationships. Unemployed people cannot be healthy in a society that values only people in paid employment, and it is very unlikely that health can be fully achieved in areas that lack basic resources such as clean water or services and facilities such as health care, transport and recreation.'

The social health of a society might be manifest in things like cohesion, cooperation and participation, but is also most evident (or not) in the gap between the most well off and the least well off in that society. The term 'sick society' is used to refer to an unhealthy society in the same way that an unhealthy individual might be described as 'sick'. An unhealthy (or sick) society will manifest greater levels of disorder and disruption, and its citizens will likely experience, for example, more loneliness and distress and greater inequality.

Epidemiologists Wilkinson and Pickett's (2009) seminal work on income inequality provided unequivocal evidence that it is linked with many health and social indicators in society, including average life expectancy, homicide rates, levels of trust, mental illness and obesity. More equal countries like those in Scandinavia have lower rates of child and adult obesity than countries that are more unequal such as the United States. Further work has reinforced the causal relationship between health and income inequality, leading Pickett and Wilkinson (2015: 316) to conclude that 'the body of evidence strongly suggests that income inequality affects population health and well-being', and that reducing the gap between the most well off and the least well off will result in better health and well-being for everyone. There is an overwhelming amount of evidence that health inequalities exist in many societies. For example, in England, work by Sir Michael Marmot and his team has shown how health inequalities have worsened since 2010 (Marmot et al., 2020), whilst a report on fuel poverty and cold homes in the UK published in 2022 highlights the unequal impact of these on people's health (Lee et al., 2022). See Box 2.4 for further details.

Box 2.4: Worsening health inequalities in England since 2010 (from Marmot et al., 2020: 3)

- Life expectancy has stalled: this has not happened since at least 1900
- Life expectancy follows the social gradient: the more deprived the area the shorter the life expectancy
- Among women in the most deprived 10 per cent of areas, life expectancy fell between 2010–12 and 2016–18
- The largest increases in life expectancy were in the least deprived 10 per cent of neighbourhoods in London; the largest decreases were in the most deprived 10 per cent of neighbourhoods in the North East
- Mortality rates increased for people aged 45–49 years.
- The amount of time people spend in poor health has increased

---

Structural violence is a term that has relevance here, referring 'to the avoidable limitations that society places on groups of people that constrain them from meeting their basic needs and achieving the quality of life that would otherwise be possible' (Lee, 2019: 123). Where people cannot access education, basic hygiene, healthcare or political power, or have restricted access to such things, structural violence is occurring. It is the structures in society (who holds power and can exercise it) that lead to structural violence. Clearly structural violence is an indicator of societal health (or the lack thereof). The important thing to note about structural violence is that, in common with health inequities, it is avoidable, preventable and correctable (Lee, 2019). Lee also refers to many different types of structural violence evident in societies worldwide; for example, healthcare disparities, increasing poverty, contemporary slavery, gender and racial disparities, and control of voting rights. In order to achieve greater societal health significant changes are needed, including the (re)distribution of power and resources. Before you read any further please take some time to do Pause for Reflection 2.1.

Pause for Reflection 2.1

Of the several different dimensions of health considered so far, which of these has greater personal resonance for you? Are there dimensions of health that hold more meaning for you? Or dimensions that do not seem relevant? Is there anything missing? What would you add and why?

Holistic health

We end this chapter by considering the notion of 'holistic' health, which Svalastog et al. (2017: 431) describe as 'an expression of wholeness'. This idea comes from holism theory, which posits that the whole is greater than its parts; holistic health therefore considers the whole person (Wills, 2023). In this sense all the dimensions of health we have considered in this chapter can be seen as parts of a whole

– as interconnected and interacting with one another, and as understood and experienced with reference to each other. We began the chapter by acknowledging that the dimensions of health under discussion are not discrete but are a theoretical, conceptual way of understanding health and health experience.

The term 'holistic health' is often used in healthcare and medical contexts, where it is frequently associated with so-called 'alternative', 'complimentary' or 'traditional' health practices which treat the person as a whole person rather than simply treating isolated symptoms: other dimensions of health are considered, not just the physical ailment or complaint that the person presents with. Holistic health is therefore a more integrated approach to health (Chronin de Chavez et al., 2005) which necessarily incorporates biological, psychological and social factors (Earle, 2007).

As we saw in Chapter 1, 'wholeness' is an idea that is reflected in lay perspectives where health is viewed as intrinsic to all other aspects of life. In the Thai context, holistic health is understood as total health or *Bai Lod*, which concerns a feeling of 'being alive with positive, active, and independent mental, physical, and spiritual functioning despite physical limitations or chronic diseases' (Detthippornpong et al., 2021: 4), as defined and experienced by older people who were homebound.

In a study on obesity among Pacific and Māori adults in South Auckland, New Zealand, holistic health was understood as involving a combination of different factors, including the physical, mental, spiritual, social and cultural (Savila et al., 2022). In their research with Indigenous communities in the United States and Canada, Walls et al. (2022: 1) argue that the concept of holistic health sits well with Indigenous notions of well-being, in which attention is given to 'the interrelationships of family, community, culture, and our environment', and that this has relevance across different cultures and in different contexts. Health then becomes about things like 'cultural identity, having a sense of connectedness to nature or family, and giving or receiving social support' (Walls et al., 2022: 1).

The concept of holistic health is also reflected in the Medicine Wheel, a North American Indigenous philosophy that reflects the equality, sacredness and interdependency of all things (Dapice, 2006). The wheel encompasses the spiritual, physical, mental and emotional, symbolizing wholeness whilst also representing cycles, seasons and change (Lavallée, 2013; Dykhuizen et al., 2022). The Medicine Wheel is rooted in Indigenous culture and traditional knowledge and takes various forms, yet the 'underlying web of meaning ... remains the same: the importance of appreciating and respecting the ongoing interconnectedness and interrelatedness of all things' (Bell, 2016: 1).

As implied by this idea, any discussion about holistic health must necessarily include the environment, incorporating planetary health, which itself requires a holistic approach, as argued by Zhang et al. (2022c) with respect to the climate change crisis. We will pick up this discussion in more detail in Chapter 8. For now, please take some time out to do Pause for Reflection 2.2.

Pause for Reflection 2.2

The latter part of this chapter has considered the notion of holistic health with specific reference to Indigenous cultures. Reflect on the social and cultural context in which you live. How is health viewed (or constructed) there? Is a holistic understanding of health evident in the structure and provision of healthcare services? If not, what do you think would need to change? What benefit might this bring to people's health experience and health outcomes?

As we have seen time and again, health is very complex and 'there are many facets that make up an individual's health' (Dykhuizen et al., 2022: 383). Holistic health is a means of appreciating and representing this complexity as well as acknowledging the intersections between the different dimensions of health. Indeed, the full extent of holistic health encompasses other dimensions of health that we have not specifically focused on in this chapter, some of which are briefly introduced in Box 2.5.

Box 2.5: Further dimensions of health (Stoewen, 2017: 861)

Intellectual health:

- Growing intellectually, maintaining curiosity about all there is to learn, valuing lifelong learning, and responding positively to intellectual challenges
- Expanding knowledge and skills while discovering the potential for sharing your gifts with others

Vocational health:

- Preparing for and participating in work that provides personal satisfaction and life enrichment that is consistent with your values, goals and lifestyle
- Contributing your unique gifts, skills and talents to work that is personally meaningful and rewarding

Financial health:

- Managing your resources to live within your means, making informed financial decisions and investments, setting realistic goals, and preparing for short-term and long-term needs or emergencies
- Being aware that everyone's financial values, needs and circumstances are unique

Case Study 2: Holistic approaches to sexual health (summarized from McDaid et al., 2019)

Sexual health is defined by the World Health Organization (2006b) as 'a state of physical, mental and social well-being in relation to sexuality. It requires a positive and respectful approach to sexuality and sexual relationships, as well as the possibility of having pleasurable and safe sexual experiences, free of coercion, discrimination and violence.' McDaid et al. (2019) carried out a qualitative study exploring understandings of holistic sexual health among men and women in deprived areas of Scotland, in the light of growing evidence for the need to have holistic approaches to promoting sexual health. The research team conducted interviews with men and women from the most deprived areas of Glasgow, Edinburgh, Dundee and three Highland towns. They found that the participants 'overwhelmingly' associated sexual health with avoiding sexually transmitted infections and unwanted pregnancies (physical health). Most of the women located their accounts of sexual health within a broader, social account of relationships that, in an ideal world, and in contrast with their everyday lives, would be based on respect and freedom from violence (social health). They expressed a desire for more positive relationships based on open communication and trust, choice, and freedom from coercion (links to mental health). In contrast, while a minority of the men were accepting of a broader definition of sexual health, most of them resisted this and put the onus to enact choices and ensure freedom from coercion on women rather than men. The research concluded that there was a disconnect between men's and women's understandings of holistic sexual health and that new efforts were needed to emphasize the breadth of sexual health. However, they acknowledged that negative underlying gender norms stood in the way of achieving this, and that interventions at individual, community and system levels would be required.

Summary

This chapter has considered different dimensions of health. As implied at the outset, this is a rather artificial way of thinking about health, since all of the dimensions are connected and interrelated with one another, and a person will experience health in all of these dimensions at the same time – as holistic health. Nevertheless, as Scriven (2017) argues, considering health in its different dimensions is a useful way of acknowledging and discussing its complexities. Using the construct of dimensions of health, it becomes possible to tease out some of its complexities and to better understand what health might mean. It should be clear by this point that health is a multidimensional concept. The next chapter will move the theoretical discussion along by exploring different models of health.

Further reading

Chinn, V., Neely, E., Shultz, S., Kruger, R., Hughes, R., Page, R. et al. (2023) Next Level Health: a holistic health and well-being program to empower New Zealand women. *Health Promotion International,* 38 (4), doi: 10.1093/heapro/daab205

Authors' summary: 'In western societies, health programs often focus on weight loss through exercise and diet to promote women's health. Such approaches disempower women by undervaluing important factors affecting their health like stress and sleep and narrow their scope for "health success". This article reports on the development of Next Level Health (NLH) that aims to help women gain greater health-related control by broadening their approach to health. The program is designed to support women to set small, achievable goals across six domains (physical activity, sleep, nutrition, eating behavior, self-care, and stress management) towards developing positive and sustainable health behaviors. Although women work with a facilitator each month to set goals, they are ultimately in control of formulating their health plans and their progression through NLH. Women can support each other by joining a community of other NLH participants through a social media group. NLH offers a novel program that is responsive to women's individual health needs and broadens their potential for health success.'

3
Models of Health

Chapter aims

- To explore western mainstream understandings of health, as represented by the biomedical model of health, and the limits of these
- To explore the social model of health and show how it challenges the biomedical model of health
- To introduce a working model of health as proposed by Green and Tones
- To explore Indigenous models of health and illustrate their depth and complexity with specific reference to the New Zealand and Canadian contexts

Introduction

This chapter provides the theoretical basis for thinking about health. The chapter will start with an exploration of Lalonde's health field concept. Several other models will then be introduced, discussed and critiqued. These include the biomedical model of health, the social model of health, the biopsychosocial model of health (Sarafino and Smith, 2022) and a 'working model of health' which brings together aspects of the preceding models (Green et al., 2019). Each model is described and outlined in detail. The chapter then moves on to consider non-western models of health as rooted in Indigenous understandings of health and well-being. These are considered in general terms before looking in some detail at Indigenous concepts of health in Māori populations in New Zealand and Indigenous people in Canada to end the discussion in this chapter.

An introduction to models of health

Why models of health? Models are a useful way to think about health and what it is/means as well as how it is experienced. Models are typically used to try to represent reality, or to make sense of something. They tend to have different component parts (sometimes referred to as constructs or variables), and attempt to show how these different parts relate to or interact with one another. Models are often presented in diagrammatic form, and diagrams have been used in this chapter to illustrate the key features of some of the models under discussion. Before you read any further, please take some time to carry out Pause for Reflection 3.1.

> **Pause for Reflection 3.1**
>
> Reflecting on what you have learned so far through reading the first chapters of this book, can you devise your own model of health? Think about the different features you would want to include in it. What would it look like? Consider the things that influence your own health and try to incorporate all the different elements in a way that makes sense to you. You could start with a list of different ideas and then group them together in some way before trying to produce a diagram of some kind.

Lalonde's health field concept

In Canada in 1974 the Lalonde Report, entitled *A New Perspective on the Health of Canadians*, was published (Lalonde, 1974). At the time, Marc Lalonde, the author of the report, was the Minister of National Health and Welfare. The report's publication was regarded by many to be a turning point in the way health was conceptualized, at least in modern times in western (or westernized) societies. It asserted that a radical change of approach was necessary in order to address health issues, highlighting the role that lifestyles play in the creation of health in wealthier countries and drawing attention to the influence of the environment (Cross et al., 2021a). Rather than a focus solely on healthcare services as being responsible for the maintenance of health, the report advocated for a new way of thinking about health. It mapped out a broader, social framework proposing that health could be improved by tackling four key factors: individual lifestyles, human biology/genetics, healthcare services and environmental influences (see Figure 3.1 and Table 3.1). This resulted in the 'health field concept'.

Lalonde contended that the physical environment (our living and working conditions) influences health and

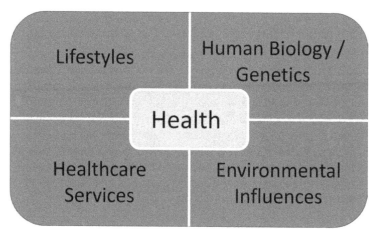

Figure 3.1: The health field concept
Source: Adapted from Lalonde (1974)

Table 3.1: Health field concept elements

Individual lifestyles	Lifestyle is considered to be the cumulation of individual decisions that affect health, and over which people have some degree of control.
Human biology/genetics	This includes physical and mental aspects of health located within the human body that are a result of basic biology and our organic make-up.
Healthcare services	This refers to the quality, quantity and arrangement of, and access to, people and resources in healthcare provision.
Environmental influences	This includes everything outside of the human body that impacts health and which people have little or no control over.

Source: Adapted from Lalonde (1974: 31–2), cited in Cross and Woodall (2024: 85–6)

experiences of health. The birth of this model signalled a move towards the prevention of ill health. The model is both simple and comprehensive (Cross and Woodall, 2024): simple in respect of having few components, yet comprehensive in the sense that it covers a wide and diverse range of factors. The health field concept is also a useful model for thinking about the determinants of health, which we will consider in more detail in Chapter 4.

The biomedical model of health

The biomedical model of health – sometimes also called the medical model (Blaxter, 2010) – has emerged from scientific understandings of the body based on its physiological mechanics and functioning. This model draws on sciences such as physiology, anatomy, pathophysiology, pharmacology, biology, histopathology and biochemistry (Scriven, 2017). It has dominated so-called western ideas about health for the last couple of centuries (Woodall and Cross, 2022), ever since the Enlightenment when, as Wills (2023: 6) states, 'in an atmosphere when everything was deemed knowable through the proper application of scientific method, the human body became a key object for the pursuit of scientific knowledge'.

The biomedical model locates health within the individual person (and specifically their body). As such it 'recognizes that individual behaviour can be a risk factor [and] it sees behaviour change as something that is in the power of the individual' (Hubley et al., 2021: 23); it therefore emphasizes individual responsibility for health (Scriven, 2017). So, it promotes a reductionist view which is a very simple, limited way of understanding health (Warwick-Booth et al., 2021) in terms of physical causes such as bacteria, germs, etc. (Tapper, 2021), often referred to as micro-causality (Cross and Woodall, 2024). In this perspective, health is conceptualized in terms of disease, pathology, disability or injury caused or created by biological or physiological means. In addition, the mind and body are seen as separate from one another, leading to ideas about mind-body dualism (Cross and Woodall, 2024) (see Figure 3.2).

The biomedical model privileges expert, professional opinions on health and focuses on the absence of disease, disability or abnormality. Therefore, if someone does not have a medically defined illness or infirmity, they are deemed

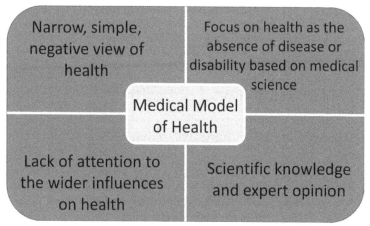

Figure 3.2: The medical model of health

to be healthy (Warwick-Booth et al., 2021). These ideas were apparent in the first two chapters, particularly in relation to the physical dimension of health discussed in Chapter 2. As we have seen, they form the basis of many contemporary understandings of what health is and have been very influential in some contexts, although not all. As Cross and Woodall (2024) argue, the biomedical model of health is 'very much in tune with modernist rational thought', and this can be seen in its domination of healthcare professional training (Wills, 2023). It is, by definition, associated with the medical profession and therefore, by implication, with the authority and power rooted in the framing of objective scientific knowledge as revealing the 'truth' about reality and experience.

Of course, the biomedical model of health has a significant role to play in the creation and maintenance of health through treatment and cure, and as such it provides the basis for many healthcare services. As Lupton (2012) argues, medicine (and the biomedical model) still has significant power. The model has been hugely influential in the treatment (and cure) of many diseases, and even in the eradication of some (for example, smallpox); however, it is not without its critics. One of the most significant criticisms of the model is that it perpetuates the idea of health as the absence of disease, because many of the indicators used to measure the existence of health are actually measuring the incidence of illness, injury and death (Hubley et al., 2021). See Box 3.1 for further criticisms.

The social model of health

The social model of health is seen by many to be the antithesis of the biomedical model in that it presents some polar-opposite ideas. It acknowledges that many different factors outside the human body influence health and it allows the complexities of health to be taken into account. These include, for example, economic, environmental, social, cultural and political factors (Warwick-Booth et al., 2021). The social model of health locates health experience within the broader context of everyday lives, not just in the individual physical body. This takes into consideration the wider structural and

---

Box 3.1: Criticisms of the biomedical model of health

- Little attention given to the wider determinants of health such as social and environmental influences (Warwick-Booth et al., 2021)
- Too simplistic; does not allow for complexity and nuance
- Promotes a negative view of health, as simply abnormality or the absence of disease (Earle, 2007)
- Expert-led, top-down orientation (Cross and Woodall, 2024)
- Promotes individual responsibility for health (Friesen, 2018)
- Focuses on pathogenic explanations for why people become ill and promotes the idea that health can only be understood through scientific means (Wills, 2023)

---

environmental factors that impact on health – for example, poverty, discrimination and inequality – and the model also incorporates issues such as sustainability (Duncan, 2013). This broader focus is one of the key things that sets the social model apart from the biomedical model (Woodall and Cross, 2022): it emphasizes what might be referred to as macro-causality in contrast to the biomedical model's focus on micro-causality (see Figure 3.3).

In the social model of health, the emphasis on responsibility for health moves from the individual to the collective (Scriven, 2017). The model also takes social interaction and social relationships into account. Social construction is key to the social model of health, with health being viewed as socially constructed (as discussed in more detail in Chapter 1). As a result, the social model privileges lay perspectives on health over expert or professional ones. It allows for consideration of differing experiences of health whilst seeking to explore why differences (in particular, inequalities) exist, and acknowledging that health is understood in various ways.

The social model has attracted some criticisms, although not as many as the biomedical model. One criticism is that it is too broad, making it not very practical in real terms.

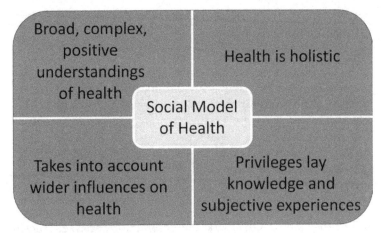

Figure 3.3: The social model of health

Another is that, rather than being set up in opposition to the biomedical model, the social model should subsume the biomedical model because science and medicine also have a part to play in subjective understandings of what health is (as demonstrated by the discussion in the previous two chapters). Earle et al. (2007) suggest that, given its breadth, the rhetoric of the social model of health is perhaps more useful. They recommend that it be used as a set of underlying values, as a set of guiding principles to inform health work, and as a set of objectives for practice. The social model offers an integrated perspective on health that encompasses all the different dimensions presented in Chapter 2. Notably, in contrast to the biomedical model, the social model views health holistically. The holistic dimension of health was discussed in the previous chapter and will feature again later in this one. Before moving on, please take some time to do Pause for Reflection 3.2.

The biopsychosocial model of health

The biopsychosocial model of health was initially proposed by psychiatrist George Engel (cited in Sarafino and Smith, 2022). As the name implies, this model is a combination of the social, the psychological and the biological attributes

Pause for Reflection 3.2

So far we have considered the biomedical model and the social model. It should be apparent by now that these are very different ways of conceptualizing health. Take some time out to summarize what you see as the main differences between the two models. Which model is more influential on the way that you view health yourself? How does this impact on your understanding and practice in relation to your own health?

of health, and it considers the interaction between these three dimensions. Social attributes of health include our social relationships, networks and communities; psychological attributes include how we think, feel and behave; whilst biological attributes include our physiological state and genetic make-up. The biopsychosocial model proposes that a person's mental state and their social capacities need to be considered alongside their physical state (Hubley et al., 2021). In addition, as Scriven (2017) argues, the model acknowledges the influence of our cultural and social environments on our health, as represented in the social dimension of the model. The advantages of the biopsychosocial model are generally agreed to be its holistic nature and its inclusion of different perspectives (Henriques, 2015). There are, however, some criticisms of it too (see Box 3.2 for details).

The biopsychosocial model is best represented by three overlapping spheres (see Figure 3.4). Health sits at the centre of the diagram, where all three spheres connect and overlap with one another, showing the influence of all three dimensions on health. In addition, the biological overlaps with the social, the social with the psychological, and the psychological with the biological.

Application of the biopsychosocial model of health to mental health and illness

Porter (2020) advocates for the use of the biopsychosocial model of health in exploring and understanding the complexities of

Box 3.2: Criticisms of the biopsychosocial model of health

According to Ghaemi (2011), the biopsychosocial model of health is:

- Too inclusive
- Too eclectic ('an unprincipled mixing of many different approaches')
- Pluralistic and reductionist

According to Henriques (2015), the biopsychosocial model of health is:

- Unscientific
- Too simplistic
- Too ambiguous, and
- The boundaries and interrelationships between the three different parts of the model are unclear

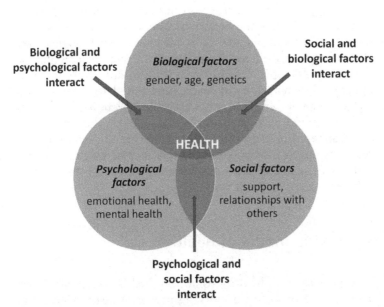

Figure 3.4: The biopsychosocial model of health
Source: Adapted from Sarafino and Smith (2022)

mental health and illness. In order to better make sense of the model it is useful to consider it in relation to mental health and illness, looking at each of the three spheres – biological, psychological and social – and their interrelations. The biological dimension of the model accounts for mental health or illness in biological terms, identifying, for example, the maintenance or disruption of chemicals in the brain, or a predisposition to experiencing mental distress due to genetic factors. In addition, certain physiological conditions or ailments – such as dementia or experiencing a stroke or brain injury – may cause symptoms of mental ill health. The psychological dimension of the model accounts for factors such as how we cope with stress and manage our emotions, how we think and behave, and our personality, all of which can influence experiences of mental health and illness. The social dimension of the model considers factors such as the impact of our relationships with other people, including our family, on our mental health, and also how culture might influence how we exhibit and interpret signs of mental health and illness, as well as systems of social support (or the lack of them). Where the biological intersects with the social this might include, for example, the effects of taking psychotropic drugs on our relationships and social interactions. Where the biological intersects with the psychological, this might include the physical and psychological side effects of prescribed medication used to treat mental illness. Some psychotropic medications, for example, can increase appetite. Likewise steroid medications used to treat several types of illness can bring undesirable psychological effects such as mood disturbances. Where the psychological and social spheres intersect this might include impacts upon family relationships as a result of life events or past trauma. Mental (ill) health sits at the very centre of the model where all three spheres overlap and intersect.

A working model of health

Two professors of health promotion, Jackie Green and Keith Tones, have proposed a working model of health that takes into account several different aspects of health (see Cross and Woodall, 2024). The model brings together many of the ideas we have discussed in this chapter in relation to other models of health, as well as ideas about dimensions of health discussed in the previous chapter. As can be seen from Figure 3.5, the model encompasses ideas about positive and negative health. The 'absence of disease' factor also acknowledges that health is experienced within a physical dimension. Positive health is conceived as well-being (which will be discussed in greater depth in Chapter 5). The working model also includes mental health, conceived in two aspects: cognitive and affective. Cognitive refers to how and what we think, while affective, in this model, covers both emotional and spiritual health. Well-being (positive health) and disease (negative health) are presented as co-existing rather than as opposite ends of a spectrum as they are commonly conceived (Cross and Woodall, 2024). This is in recognition of the fact that a person may be physically unwell yet experience good levels of subjective well-being, or, conversely, physically robust yet suffering mentally, emotionally or socially.

Importantly, the working model also takes into account health at the individual level and at the social level, recognizing the salience of both. At the individual level the model emphasizes the importance of independence, interpersonal

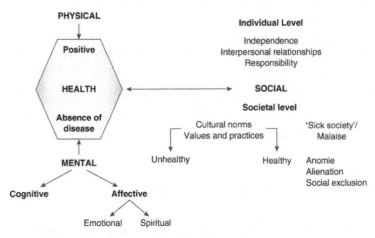

Figure 3.5: A working model of health
Source: Cross and Woodall (2024)

Table 3.2: Three main aspects of individual social health

Independence	A socially mature individual acts with greater independence and autonomy than a relatively immature individual.
Interpersonal relationships	A socially healthy individual is characterized by the capacity to relate to a number of significant others and cooperate with them.
Responsibility	A person who is socially mature accepts responsibility for health.

Source: Adapted from Cross and Woodall (2024: 16)

relationships and responsibility for health (see Table 3.2). At the social level it recognizes the complexity of the social dimension of health, taking into account how health and health experience are influenced by the cultural and social norms, values and practices which inform people's ideas about what they understand to be 'healthy' and 'unhealthy'.

The working model also considers the health of society as a whole and incorporates ideas around the 'sick society' (discussed in more detail in the previous chapter). Finally, again with reference to the health of society, the model includes the constructs of anomie (social divisions and lack of solidarity), alienation and social exclusion, recognizing that an unhealthy society will manifest in these ways. The working model of health was presented as a work in progress and as a challenge to the dichotomous biomedical and social models of health. In bringing many aspects of health together it provides a more comprehensive account that better represents the complexities of health within a single framework.

Indigenous models of health

There is a significant amount of research showing that Indigenous populations across the world suffer greater health inequalities than their non-Indigenous counterparts (Flood and Rohloff, 2018). It has been argued that these inequalities can be tackled (in part at least) by gaining a better appreciation of Indigenous perspectives on health (McIntosh et al., 2021; Wilson et al., 2021). We consider Indigenous perspectives here with a note of caution – it is not possible to go into the depth that is needed to fully appreciate all the nuances and richness in these perspectives; consequently, as Wilson et al. (2021) rightly point out, there is a risk of oversimplifying complex ideas. Nevertheless, bearing that in mind we can say that, in general, Indigenous views of health tend to privilege community over the individual, and recognize the connectedness of people with each other, their natural environment and their history, in deep and intricate ways that the models we have discussed so far tend to overlook. The environment (social, physical, etc.) is considered in some of the models, such as the social model and the working model, but not in the sense in which it is recognized in many Indigenous models of health. Likewise, the social nature of health is reflected in some of the other models, but the concept of community is not emphasized in the same way as it is in Indigenous models of health. In Indigenous perspectives, health is viewed as 'a balance that is achieved within the physical, emotional, spiritual and mental domains of individual and community life' (Kelley, 2010: 5). There is also evidence to show that Indigenous perspectives on health promote more sustainable ways of living and being. In this section we will explore several different Indigenous models of health, drawing on understandings from two different countries (New Zealand and Canada), and showing how westernized models (particularly the biomedical model) are oftentimes inconsistent with these and, sometimes, even in direct conflict (Kelley, 2010).

Māori models of health (Aotearoa/New Zealand)

For the Māori of Aotearoa/New Zealand, health is inextricably linked with Indigenous culture and with the landscape (McIntosh et al., 2021). Wilson et al. (2021) identified four overarching themes within Māori perspectives: health and well-being; connectedness (*whanaungatanga*); relationship building (*whakawhanaungatanga*); and sociopolitical health contexts (colonization, urbanization, racism and marginalization). They observe that, for Māori, health is a 'holistic and relational concept' (Wilson et al., 2021: 3539).

Māori culture has a holistic worldview in which connections to landscape (physical spaces), to the natural world and to ancestral roots are very important (McIntosh et al., 2021). Similarly to other contexts, the arrival of Europeans severely disrupted traditional ways of Māori life as land was taken away from them, resulting in their separation from each other, from tradition and from the land itself. This had devastating effects on health experience and health outcomes for Māori populations. Contemporary understandings of health in Māori culture are rooted in pre-colonial history, where family, community and the land had huge significance in terms of identity and belonging. McIntosh et al. (2021) present three different Māori models of health, which are summarized in Table 3.3.

Whilst differently conceptualized, the three Māori models of health have many things in common, foremost of which is the (inter)connectedness of different dimensions of health and the importance of balance between them. Another theme is the importance of land or the physical environment. In Māori culture people are viewed as being inextricably linked to the landscape, which significantly influences health: 'Historically, Māori have always had a strong relationship with land (mother Earth – *Papatūānuku*) as it shapes the way in which they express their cultural, spiritual, emotional, physical and social well-being', and Māori possess what is described as a 'reverence' for the natural environment not always seen in more modern cultures (McIntosh et al., 2021: 150). McIntosh et al. concluded that culture, health and landscape are all interconnected in Māori concepts of well-being. Māori models of health illustrate how health is a sociocultural construct and, as Wilson et al. (2021) argue, show how crucial it is to appreciate differences in perspectives, worldviews and cultural understandings of health.

Indigenous communities in Canada

Like other contexts where Indigenous people have been colonialized and marginalized, the Indigenous communities

Table 3.3: Three Māori models of health

Te Whare Tapa Whā (the four cornerstones)	This model uses the analogy of a house to represent the importance of balance. Each of the four walls of the house represents a different dimension of health. The first, *taha tinana*, is the physical body; the second, *taha wairua*, is the spiritual realm; the third, *taha whanau*, is family and community; and the fourth, *taha hinengaro*, is mental health. 'All four elements are interwoven and interact to support a strong and healthy person' (McIntosh et al., 2021: 147). Any imbalance between or within the four walls will lead to poor health. The concept of harmony is also important in this model – people must live in accord with others and with the spiritual realm.
Te Pae Māhutonga (Southern Cross constellation)	Named after a constellation of six stars seen in the southern hemisphere, this model brings together six elements of health promotion. Four stars form the cross for which the constellation is named. These represent cultural identity (*mauriora*), the physical environment (*waiora*), healthy lifestyle (*toiora*) and participation in society (*te orange*). The two pointer stars represent leadership (*ngā manukura*) and autonomy (*te mana whakahaere*).
Te Wheke (the octopus)	In this model the different body parts of the octopus represent different aspects of health. The head represents the family (*te whanau*), the eyes represent the overall well-being of the individual and family (*waiora*), and each of the eight tentacles represents different aspects of health as follows:

1. Spirituality (*wairuatanga*)
2. The mind (*hinengaro*)
3. Physical well-being (*taha tinana*)
4. Extended family (*whanaungatanga*)
5. Life force in people and objects (*mauri*)
6. Unique identity of individuals and family (*mana ake*)
7. Breath of life from forebears (*hā a koro ma, a kui ma*)
8. The open and healthy expression of emotion (*whatumanawa*)

All of these aspects of health are closely entwined with one another, representing 'the close relationships that exist between each health dimension' (McIntosh et al., 2021: 149). This model emphasizes the inextricable connections between the health of a person, their family and their wider community.

of Canada suffer a greater burden of ill health as compared to the majority population of non-Indigenous Canadians (Kelley, 2010). Indigenous perspectives on health have been relatively neglected in mainstream health service provision, leading to inequalities in health for the Indigenous minority (Fijal and Beagan, 2019). In a review of the literature on Indigenous perspectives on health in Canada, Fijal and Beagan (2019) found three main themes – balance, community and land. Whilst acknowledging variations in Indigenous cultures, they observe how health is conceived as a balance between different elements of health – physical, emotional, mental and spiritual. Physical health included ideas about a healthy diet, linked to traditional foodstuffs, and about exercise, linked to traditional activities such as hunting. Emotional health included ideas about positive support from others and staying busy. Mental health included ideas about making 'good choices', taking personal responsibility and having a positive attitude, as well as being connected to the land. Spiritual health included ideas about being connected to everything, a belief in a higher power, and engaging in traditional practices, customs and ceremonies that reflect a respect for Elders, who 'play an important role in the transmission of knowledge and practices' (Fijal and Beagan, 2019: 224). The connection between culture and the land was also very apparent, as was connecting with cultural heritage.

The second key theme, community, highlights the importance of connecting with others and the value of relationship and communication. Community, including intergenerational connection, is viewed as essential to health. This is also manifest through ideas of reciprocity and helping other people. Finally, the theme of land demonstrates how our relationship to the earth and its flora and fauna is also viewed as essential to health. The sacredness of certain physical places linked with healing, spirituality, family and tradition is entwined with notions of balance and well-being. Fijal and Beagan's (2019) research provides an overview of several Indigenous models of health. As Smylie and Anderson (2006: 604) state, 'although Indigenous models of health are diverse, they generally differ from non-Indigenous biomedical models in that they consider

Case Study 3: Models of health and disability

Medical model of disability
The medical model of disability views disability as a problem with the individual person resulting from a physical impairment or condition. For example, if a wheelchair user wants to access an ice cream shop but there is no ramp, the medical model says that the person's inability to enter the shop is due to their impairment. The problem is the person's impairment, not the building's lack of access.

Social model of disability
The social model of disability views disability as a problem with society caused by the structural barriers that people living with disabilities face in their everyday lives, for example in terms of exclusion and discrimination. Disability is viewed in terms of subjective experience, not as pathological. If a wheelchair user wants to access an ice cream shop but there is no ramp, the social model says they are disabled only by the lack of a ramp to the building, which removes access, independence and opportunity.

Biopsychosocial model of disability
The biopsychosocial model of disability takes into account the medical model and the social model while recognizing that psychological factors also need to be taken into account. Psychological factors include things like coping mechanisms, thoughts and feelings. Utilizing a biopsychosocial model of disability allows for a more holistic approach in which the whole person is considered.

Sources: The Nora Project, thenoraproject.ngo; Disability Nottingham, disabilitynottinghamshire.org.uk; Physiopedia, physio-pedia.com

the health of the whole community and its surrounding environment'.*

Summary

This chapter has considered several models of health in some detail. However, the content of the chapter is not exhaustive. For example, we have not considered the ecological model of health. This will be discussed in the final chapter of the book. In this chapter we have examined different models of health, some of which have commonalities. The working model of health provides the most comprehensive 'western' model of health and demonstrates its complexities more thoroughly than do the preceding models discussed here. However, Indigenous models of health offer more diverse, richer conceptualizations of health, as we latterly discussed in relation to Indigenous perspectives from New Zealand and Canada. A closer consideration of models of health, as seen in this chapter, moves us towards thinking about what determines health. Lalonde's (1974) health field concept provides a firm foundation for exploring determinants of health. The next chapter will examine these in greater depth.

Further reading

Sarafino, E.P. and Smith, T.W. (2022) *Health Psychology: Biopsychosocial Interactions.* 10th edition. Chichester, Wiley.

This popular, accessible book is now in its tenth edition. It provides comprehensive content relating to the biopsychosocial

---

* Note that Indigenous cultures in Canada (and elsewhere) are not homogeneous. There are variations in dialects, culture and traditional practices. What Indigenous people do have in common, however, is their shared history of collective trauma, which for many continues to the present day, as is evident in the significant health inequalities that exist and the lack of parity in terms of access to healthcare services, education and employment.

model of health, drawing on a range of international research and case studies. Although focused on health psychology and written by psychologists, this book is very relevant not just to the discussion in this chapter, but for other content elsewhere in *What is Health?*

4
Determinants of Health

Chapter aims

- To explore what is meant by the term 'determinants of health'
- To introduce, describe and apply key models of social determinants of health
- To critically consider health inequality and inequity, and issues of structure and agency
- To propose some strategies for tackling the wider determinants of health

Introduction

This chapter considers what determines health. It starts by exploring what is meant by the term 'determinants of health' and then moves on to introduce two models of social determinants of health – Dahlgren and Whitehead's (1991) classic 'rainbow' model, as well as the more contemporary framework from the Commission on the Social Determinants of Health (Solar and Irwin, 2010). The social determinants of health are discussed in relation to these two models. This includes consideration of structural determinants of health, such as social class, gender and commercial determinants of health. The chapter examines health inequalities and inequity and draws on a range of international research to illustrate how health experience is inconsistent between, and within, countries in our modern world. This includes some discussion about responsibility for health as well as issues of structure and agency. The seminal work of Sir Michael Marmot and his team is considered in some detail in this chapter, which ends with some final thoughts about how the social determinants of health might be tackled in order to create fairer health outcomes for all.

What are determinants of health?

Determinants of health might also be described as 'influences on health' (Wills, 2023: 17). When we talk about what determines or influences health, we need to take into consideration everything that has been discussed in the first three chapters of this book – how we define health, the different dimensions of health, and how we conceptualize health. It is not possible to think about what determines health without recognition of these factors. By now you should have a very good appreciation of the complexity of health. Any discussion about what determines health is also necessarily complex.

Determinants of health are numerous and intricately connected. There are many different factors that influence our health, our health experience and our health outcomes. As Scriven (2017) argues, the combination of these different factors will shape our health, whatever we consider health to be. Recent research on the British public's ideas about what influences their health shows that people tend to focus only on two things – individual behaviour and the ability to access healthcare services (Kane et al., 2022). However, although important, we know that health is determined by much more than these two things. Lalonde's (1974) health field concept, introduced in Chapter 3, recognizes that health is influenced by four factors – biology and genetics, lifestyle, healthcare provision and our environment. This model has since been superseded by more complex ones. Later in this chapter we will consider some of these models in more detail, but here we will focus on some specific determinants of health, starting with the commonly used term 'social determinants of health'. Before reading any further take some time out to do Pause for Reflection 4.1.

Pause for Reflection 4.1

What determines your health? Think about what (and who) influences it and how. You could also think about someone other than yourself – a relative or client perhaps. What determines or influences their health? It might help to think about a typical day and what happens to you from the moment you open your eyes in the morning to the moment you go to bed at night. No doubt you will come up with a long list of different factors!

Social determinants of health

Social determinants of health encompass several different factors such as our socioeconomic status and our gender. Wills (2023: 17) defines social determinants of health as 'economic and social factors (e.g. income, social class and gender) that have a profound effect on health. These differences are not natural but are created and maintained by social and economic policies and legislation.' A key point worth reiterating here is that social determinants of health are not inevitable but come into existence because of different structures in society. This idea is supported by Kane et al. (2022: 4) (and many others), who argue, in the UK context, that 'factors such as housing, education and employment are pivotal in shaping individual opportunities to be healthy and play a stronger role in [creating] and maintaining good health than access to the National Health Service'. Among the many social determinants of health, we will focus here on social class and gender.

Social class

Social class is about the position we hold in society and is often expressed in terms of a hierarchy linked to wealth, with the wealthiest people at the top and the poorest at the bottom. Social class has also been conceptualized in relation to types of employment. For example, in the UK the Registrar General's classification is based on job role as follows:

Social Class I – Professional
Social Class II – Intermediate
Social Class IIIN – Skilled non-manual
Social Class IIIM – Skilled manual
Social Class IV – Semi-skilled manual
Social Class V – Unskilled manual

Of course, employment is directly linked to income and education levels as well. The limits of the Registrar General's classification have been recognized, although it is still widely used. In the British context, Savage et al. (2013) proposed an alternative classification that considers other forms of capital (such as social and cultural capital), not just economic capital. This includes seven categories as follows:

1. Elite (e.g. barristers and judges)
2. Established middle class (e.g. police officers, teachers)
3. Technical middle class (e.g. pharmacists, engineers)
4. New affluent workers (e.g. sales and retail assistants)
5. Traditional working class (e.g. electrical technicians)
6. Emergent service workers (e.g. chefs)
7. Precariat (e.g. cleaners)

Given that this categorization is specific to the British context it may not be immediately transferable to other countries. However, social class impacts on health in many ways. There is consistent and indisputable evidence that, in general, people from lower socioeconomic backgrounds experience worse health. For example, Williams et al. (2022: npn) note how 'lower socioeconomic groups tend to have a higher prevalence of higher-risk health behaviours, worse access to care and less opportunity to lead healthy lives than higher socioeconomic groups'.

Gender

Gender, as differentiated from biological sex, is an important social construct that influences health and health experience. Research carried out in the Asia-Pacific region into gender inequalities in health and well-being over the first two decades of life mirrored what is already known: that gender inequalities emerge in childhood, continuing through adolescence and into adulthood (Kennedy et al., 2022). This research, drawing on data from forty low- and middle-income countries in the region, revealed significant comparative disadvantage for girls and young women in relation to several factors, such as sexual and reproductive health and intimate-partner violence. It also found that boys and young men experience higher mortality due to unintentional injury, interpersonal violence, suicide, drug abuse and harmful levels of alcohol consumption and smoking (Kennedy et al., 2022). Inequalities in health between men and women can be explained by the social construction of masculinity and femininity, which (in patri-archal societies at least) generally affords greater power to men compared to women. This also results in socially prescribed ways of being and behaving for men and women that can have either a positive or a negative impact on health. As Woodall and Cross (2022) argue, the mechanisms involved in this are complex; however, evidence suggests that, whilst women tend to live longer than men, they also tend to spend more of that time in ill health in comparison. In the UK for example, the average time spent in poor health is 19.1 years for women, compared with an average of 16.1 years for men (Farand, 2017). One explanation for this is that women suffer more depression and mental health issues than men. One final example is access to healthcare services. There is a substantial amount of research evidencing gendered inequalities resulting from sexism and unconscious gender bias in healthcare systems, which have a negative impact on health experience and health outcomes (Alcalde-Rubio et al., 2020). This is a common pattern across all countries.

Social class and gender are just two social determinants of health. Others include ethnicity, race, sexuality, education, income, employment and housing – in short, all the conditions of the 'environments where people are born, live, learn, work, play, worship and age that affect a wide range of health, functioning, and quality-of-life outcomes and risks' (Healthy People 2030, 2020: npn). Healthy People 2030 groups the social determinants of health into five domains: economic stability, education access and quality, healthcare access and quality, neighbourhood and built environment, and social and community context. See Box 4.1 for some further examples of social determinants of health.

Box 4.1: Examples of social determinants of health (Healthy People 2030, 2020)

- Safe housing, transportation and neighbourhoods
- Racism, discrimination and violence
- Education, job opportunities and income
- Access to nutritious foods and physical activity opportunities
- Polluted air and water
- Language and literacy skills

Commercial determinants of health

Commerce (the exchange of goods and services) has only really been appreciated as a determinant of health within the past ten years or so (Lacy-Nichols et al., 2023), based on a recognition of the fact that the private sector is driven by profit margins and that this can, at times, cause conflict with the pursuit of health: 'commercial actors, particularly large, multinational commercial actors, have the social, economic, and political gravity to shape the world in ways health departments and even entire national governments cannot' (Maani et al., 2023: 4). Commercial determinants of health are complex, multidimensional, upstream factors that shape patterns of consumption which, in turn, can have a negative impact on health experience and health outcomes (Knai and Savona, 2023). Corporate strategy can influence government policy, whilst advertising strategies influence individual consumer choices. Although there is as yet no agreed definition of commercial determinants of health (Lacy-Nichols et al., 2023), there is increasing recognition that they play a crucial role in the existence of health inequalities.

Technology as a determinant of health

Recent rapid changes in technology have had a significant impact on health. For example, the impact of social media on health outcomes is becoming more evident. Social media can have positive and negative influences on health, from the promotion of healthy or unhealthy behaviours (and products) to the positive or negative impact engagement with social media can have on mental and emotional health (Vassallo et al., 2021). In 2012, writing about twenty-first-century determinants of health, Ilona Kickbusch, a political scientist best known for her work on health promotion and global health, pointed out that technology had developed in significant ways over the previous decade. We have seen further rapid technological changes over the last ten years as well, and will continue to do so. Kickbusch (2012) highlighted what she saw as the three key twenty-first-century determinants of health: unsustainable lifestyles, the flow of people and the hurry virus. See Box 4.2 for more information about these.

Kickbusch's ideas perhaps reflect the priorities of the global north for the most part. In the decade that has passed since she wrote the editorial in question the world has continued to change, and the global COVID-19 pandemic has demonstrated how it can do so very quickly indeed, along with our lived experience of it. Take some time out to do Pause for Reflection 4.2.

In the next section we will consider different models of determinants of health, starting with the 'rainbow model'.

Box 4.2: Kickbusch's (2012: 6) three key twenty-first-century determinants of health

Unsustainable lifestyles
Kickbusch argued that many health challenges are related to unsustainable lifestyles and unsustainable production and consumption patterns, suggesting that the obesity epidemic and the global system of food production, distribution, consumption and waste are symptoms of this.

The flow of people
Kickbusch commented on the increased movement of people internationally through tourism, migration, mobility and displacement, and argued that, at the time, the full impact of this on health had not been realized.

The hurry virus
The hurry virus – a term coined by Tranter, cited in Kickbusch (2012: 6) – refers to 'the feeling of constantly having to rush', which affects children as well as adults. Kickbusch observed that several factors contribute to this, including urbanization, modern media and new forms of working, all of which contribute to time pressure, increased stress, anxiety and depression, as well as poor diets and a lack of physical activity.

Pause for Reflection 4.2

What did you make of the 'hurry virus' idea? Does it resonate with you and your life, and with those around you? Do you find yourself feeling like you constantly have to rush? What causes that feeling? What factors of modern-day life lead people to feel that way? Do you think it is worse now than a decade ago? If so, why?

Dahlgren and Whitehead's (1991) model of health determinants

Based on its diagrammatic form, Dahlgren and Whitehead's model of health determinants is sometimes referred to as the 'rainbow model', as it will be here. Each concentric layer of the rainbow represents different influences on health, starting with the factors at the centre of it – those that we cannot change, such as our age (however much we try to!), our genetic inheritance and our biological sex as determined by our chromosomes. The next layer represents our lifestyle – the behaviours and practices that we engage in (or not). These might include things like what we eat, how we cope with and manage stress, and how much alcohol we consume or the amount and type of physical activity we engage in (or not). Moving further outwards, the next layer of the rainbow represents our social and community networks. This includes our friends and family. The support (or lack thereof) we receive from other people has a large bearing on our health and health experience. The penultimate layer represents our living and working conditions. The model refers to the following factors in this regard: agriculture and food production, education, work environment, unemployment, water and sanitation, healthcare services and housing. The final layer of the rainbow represents general socioeconomic, cultural and environmental conditions (see Figure 4.1).

Several decades have passed since the rainbow model was first conceptualized, but Warwick-Booth et al. (2021) recognize its continued saliency given its several strengths, including its relative simplicity, the ability to apply it to different issues and contexts, and the way it demonstrates that individual choices and behaviour have comparatively little influence on health. However, the model can be criticized on several counts. It is now over three decades since it was introduced and the world has changed a lot since then, particularly in terms of technology, digitization and globalization. See Box 4.3 for details on the limitations of the rainbow model.

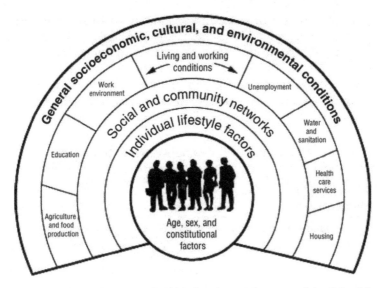

Figure 4.1: Dahlgren and Whitehead's rainbow model of health determinants

Source: Dahlgren and Whitehead (1991)

Box 4.3: Limitations of the rainbow model (adapted from Warwick-Booth et al., 2021: 280–2)

- It is more descriptive than explanatory, does not provide detail about the (inter)relationships between the different influences on health, and does not sufficiently demonstrate the complexities of determinants of health
- It lacks consideration of global, political, commercial and historical determinants of health
- The relationships between the different layers of the rainbow are more complicated than the model suggests
- The natural environment is not specifically considered; this is ever more important as we see the impact of climate change on planetary and human health
- The life course is not considered as a determinant of health, nor is social and geographical mobility

In recognition of some of the limitations of the rainbow model, Dahlgren and Whitehead revisited it in 2007, suggesting that it might be viewed as an 'interdependent system for improving health and reducing health hazards' and that the four outer layers of the model could be used to inform policy intervention to tackle inequities in health (Dahlgren and Whitehead, 2007: 13). See Table 4.1 for

Table 4.1: Application of the rainbow model to malaria

Rainbow layer (starting from the middle of the model and working outwards)	Example determinants
Age, sex and constitutional factors	Age is a risk factor for malaria – young children are more vulnerable. Pregnant women are also more vulnerable.
Individual lifestyle factors	Some individual behaviours increase or decrease susceptibility to infection, such as taking preventative measures (using insecticide-treated nets [ITNs] and insect repellent, taking prophylactics and seeking early treatment when sick).
Social and community networks	The influence of other people on help-seeking behaviour and engaging in preventative measures is important. Power dynamics in families can affect who has access to ITNs and access to treatment when sick.
Living and working conditions	Water storage and vector control are significant factors in reducing mosquito breeding sites. Access (or the lack of it) to healthcare services for quick and effective treatment once infected will influence health outcomes.
General socioeconomic, cultural and environmental conditions	Poverty and socioeconomic disadvantage are directly linked to health outcomes for malaria, for example in terms of being able to afford ITNs and treatment once sick.

an application of the model to the issue of malaria, where various determinants are considered in relation to this significant global health challenge.

The rainbow model was further developed by Barton and Grant (2006) to take into account the major role that the environment plays in determining our health and well-being. Barton and Grant's model will be discussed in more detail in Chapter 8.

The Commission on the Social Determinants of Health (CSDH) framework (Solar and Irwin, 2010)

The World Health Organization has led developments examining the social determinants of health. In 2010 the Commission on the Social Determinants of Health conceptual framework was published, to further understanding (Solar and Irwin, 2010). As can be seen from Figure 4.2, this framework is a much more complex representation of determinants of health than Dahlgren and Whitehead's rainbow model.

The main purposes of the framework are, firstly, to try to make sense of the many complex factors that influence and impact on health (Warwick-Booth and Cross, 2018), and, secondly, to examine different levels of causation, highlighting the conditions of daily life which result from the distribution of power through the creation of social hierarchies (Solar and Irwin, 2010). The framework brings together political, economic, ecological and psychosocial factors. As Solar and Irwin (2010: 4) state: 'a key aim of the framework is to highlight the difference between levels of causation, distinguishing between the mechanisms by which social hierarchies are created, and the conditions of daily life which then result'. There are, therefore, two distinct parts to the framework: one that considers the *structural determinants of health*, and one that considers the *intermediary determinants of health*. Structural determinants of health refer to social status or position, as indicated by factors such as social class, income, level of education, gender, occupation

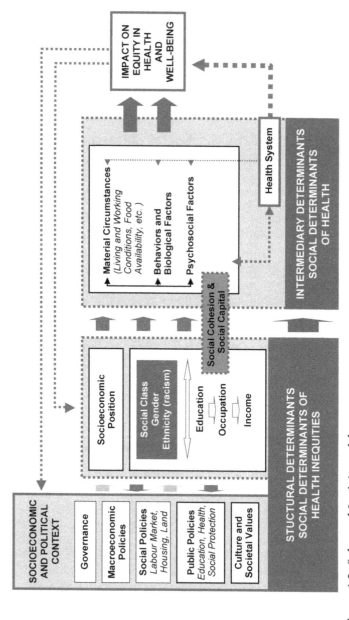

Figure 4.2: Solar and Irwin's model
Source: Solar and Irwin (2010)

and ethnicity. Intermediary determinants of health refer to material circumstances, behavioural and biological factors, psychosocial factors and the health system. See Box 4.4 for further information.

Box 4.4: Intermediary determinants of health (Solar and Irwin, 2010: 6)

Material circumstances include factors such as housing and neighbourhood quality, consumption potential (e.g. the financial means to buy healthy food, warm clothing, etc.), and the physical work environment.

Psychosocial circumstances include psychosocial stressors, stressful living circumstances and relationships, and social support and coping styles (or the lack thereof).

Behavioural and biological factors include nutrition, physical activity and tobacco and alcohol consumption, which are distributed differently among different social groups. Biological factors also include genetic determinants (and ageing).

The three key determinants of twenty-first-century health presented earlier in Box 4.2 are, as Kickbush (2012: 6) argued, 'intricately linked ... to the political determinants of health'. Thus the political context features prominently in the CSDH model in acknowledgement that power is a major determinant of health: governance, economic policies, social policies and public policies are accounted for in the CSDH framework. This includes issues of macroeconomic, social and public policy. Culture and societal values, social cohesion and social capital also feature in the model. The arrows in the framework represent the relationships between the different concepts, including the strong connections between the structural determinants and the intermediary determinants that result, demonstrating both direct and indirect causation. In addition, the impact of the socio-economic and political context on socioeconomic position is laid bare.

Solar and Irwin's framework highlights the importance of structural and political determinants of health. Later in this chapter we will consider structure as a determinant of health in more detail, but it is appropriate here to think about the political determinants of health in relation to this framework. Politics is to do with power and, as stated earlier, power is a key determinant of health. Those with less power tend to have worse health and less opportunity or capacity to take control over their own lives. As Solar and Irwin (2010) argue, we need to understand how power operates in order to tackle health inequities, and tackling these is a political process requiring political will. One of the most important factors for health is the provision of a welfare state and distributive policies (or the lack of such provision). Thus, the role and provision of the health system (and access to it) are included as a key component in the framework. (For further detail about the CSDH framework see Solar and Irwin, 2010.)

Health inequality and inequity

Inequality and inequity are not the same. Box 4.5 provides useful definitions of health inequalities and inequity, illustrating how such inequalities are far from inevitable and that inequity is concerned with a lack of justice. Clearly both are inextricably linked.

Box 4.5: Health inequalities and inequity – definitions (Wills, 2023: 17 and 21)

Health inequalities: 'avoidable and unfair differences in health status between groups of people who are united by their shared socioeconomic status or gender rather than by any health-related attributes, for example, medical conditions such as diabetes'

Inequity: A lack of equity or fairness. Health inequity is avoidable, unjust and unfair.

There is a substantial amount of evidence that inequalities in health exist both within and between countries. Inequalities in health are those that occur because of social and economic factors (Woodall and Cross, 2022). Hilary Graham (2009), a sociologist and professor of health sciences, identifies three types of health inequality as follows:

- Health differences between individuals
- Health differences between population groups
- Health differences between different groups based on the social position they occupy

There are several explanations for the existence of health inequalities, but we are not going to discuss those in detail here because, however they are explained, health inequalities exist. There is unequivocal evidence for them at regional, national and global levels – as will be demonstrated by the discussion in this chapter. Using even the crudest measures of health – those which view health as the absence of disease – we can see stark differences in life expectancy within countries. The United Kingdom, for example, has seen a general decline in population health over the past few years as well as a widening of health inequalities. In England, increases in average life expectancy have slowed down, and they declined further due to the impact of the COVID-19 pandemic (Iacobucci, 2021). In addition, 'there are also large differences in life expectancy and healthy life expectancy between the most and least deprived areas of the country' (British Medical Association, 2022).

Using the same crude measures, we can make comparisons between countries which reveal stark contrasts indicative of gross inequalities. For example, the most recent data shows that average life expectancy in some of the wealthiest countries far exceeds that in the least well off. According to estimates from the United Nations Population Division (2023), as of early 2023, the average life expectancy of the world's population was 73.2 years, with females living, on average, a few years longer than males. However, if we look more closely at individual countries, there are huge differences. Hong Kong and Japan had the highest average at just over 85 years, whilst Sierra Leone, Nigeria, Lesotho, Chad and the Central African Republic had the lowest – all around 54 or 55 years.

People in wealthier countries, then, tend to live longer. However, the picture is not a straightforward one. The countries that tend to have better health are those where the gap between the most well off and the least well off is smaller. This is supported by the work of Wilkinson and Pickett (2009; see also Pickett and Wilkinson, 2015), who demonstrated that societies in which the gap was greatest had the worst health outcomes on a range of indicators, including mental health, homicide and obesity. In terms of mental health, countries with greater income disparities have a higher prevalence of depression, anxiety and substance misuse (WHO, 2022). Inequality does not just hurt the most vulnerable in society; it also impacts on everyone across the socioeconomic spectrum (Marmot, 2010; Marmot et al., 2020). Using subjective measures of health, people in more egalitarian societies tend to report better health. Steckermeier and Delhey's (2019) study of thirty European countries found that people in countries with higher levels of social trust and self-expression had fewer feelings of inferiority (evidence of a more egalitarian culture), whilst there was more widespread individual blame for poverty in more inegalitarian countries. Furthermore, the authors found that this egalitarian culture mattered not just for the subjective lived experience of the lowest-income groups but right across the different income levels up to the topmost tier. Using subjective measures of health such as happiness and well-being reveals different patterns as well. We will discuss these in more detail in Chapters 5 and 6.

Structure and agency

The importance of structural determinants of health was highlighted earlier in this chapter in relation to Solar and Irwin's (2010) model of the social determinants of health. In this context, structure is used as a sociological term and is a noun. The Open Education Sociology Dictionary (2023: npn) defines structure as 'the complex and stable framework of society that influences all individuals or groups through the relationship between institutions (e.g. economy, politics, religion) and social practices (e.g. behaviours, norms and values)'. The structures themselves are not visible, but the impacts of them are. In the CSDH framework, key structural factors include things like income, education, occupation, social class, gender and race/ethnicity. Here, 'structural mechanisms' are those that generate stratification and social class divisions in society and that define individual socio-economic positions within hierarchies of power, prestige and access to resources. These mechanisms are 'rooted in the key institutions and processes of the socioeconomic and political context' (Solar and Irwin, 2010: 6).

As stated earlier in this chapter, power is a key determinant of health. It is replicated and reproduced through various mechanisms, including social institutions and practices. Those with power do better in terms of health than those who are relatively powerless. As such, Kreiger (2008) argues that structures of agency need to be considered, as well as the operation of power at different levels and the impact that this has on health. Agency is another sociological term and refers to the extent to which a person is able to make their own decisions, take action and be responsible for themselves. Agency can therefore be constrained or given opportunity depending on structure.

The structure/agency debate gives rise to questions about who is responsible for health – the individual or the state. A study of the British public showed that many people consistently point to the individual as being responsible for maintaining their own health and living healthy lives; however, during the COVID-19 pandemic the emphasis on responsibility for health shifted more to government (Kane et al., 2022). There is certainly a limit to what an individual person can do to improve their own health, given that it is affected by so many social determinants. Behaviour is viewed by many to be a key determinant of health (Tapper, 2021), and it is commonly known that many chronic diseases, such as cardiovascular disease and various cancers, have an element of behavioural risk. However, generally, people are more likely to engage in unhealthy behaviours if they are socially and economically disadvantaged (Oleribe et al.,

2018). So, behaviour cannot be viewed in isolation. Our environment influences the actions and behaviours we engage in (or not) at an individual level. Social factors such as cultural norms, beliefs and values also influence behaviour (Schoon and Krumwiede, 2022).

It should be apparent by now that the persistence of health inequalities and inequity is largely down to the social structures within society that operate to privilege some people over others. As Wills (2023) argues, inequalities in health exist because of structural inequalities. The causes of these are, almost without exception, political. While there are, as we acknowledged earlier, biological and behavioural determinants of health operating at the individual level, the greatest determinants of health are social. There is therefore a limit to the amount of control a person will have over their health. Much of our health experience is determined by factors that lie outside of our power. Although the rise in non-communicable diseases has led to a focus on individual lifestyles and risk factors, it is the wider, social determinants of health that influence the choices we are able to make at the personal level. (See the Case Study later in this chapter for a more in-depth exploration of this in relation to fuel poverty and cold homes.)

Kane et al. (2022) distinguish between individualistic and ecological 'strains of thought' about health (see Box 4.6). Both strains of thought can be linked to ideas about agency and structure. Whilst they are interlinked to some extent, they represent very different worldviews. An individualistic perspective emphasizes individual agency and the capacity to act to be healthy, whilst an ecological perspective focuses on the structural factors that influence, create and maintain health.

As Solar and Irwin (2010: 5) argue, 'the central role of power in the understanding of social pathways and mechanisms means that tackling the social determinants of health inequities is a political process that engages both the agency of disadvantaged communities and the responsibility of the state'. Colonization is an example of this in terms of the impact imperialism has had (and continues to have) on the intersection of other structural factors such as gender, race, sexuality and class. Dykhuizen et al. (2022) highlight the

Box 4.6: Individualistic and ecological 'strains of thought' (Kane et al., 2022: 9)

Individualistic – an individualistic strain of thought assigns a central role to individual choice and willpower. It promotes individual-level responsibility for the choices people make, emphasizing the use of their own internal resources and experiences, and highly prizing a sense of control.

Ecological – the ecological strain of thought sees health, at least in part, as a product of social and environmental influences. It views the conditions in which we live, work and grow as crucial to our ability to stay healthy. Within this strain of thought it is easier to see the multiple conditions necessary to enable health, from cheap healthy food promoted on the shelves to good employment opportunities which allow people to live well.

inequalities in health experienced by Indigenous communities in Canada which resulted from colonial and heteropatriarchal rule and which persist in modern-day healthcare systems. This is a pattern that can be seen in other countries with similar colonial histories (Schoon and Krumwiede, 2022). As Dykhuizen et al. (2022: 385) point out: 'it is well documented that the experience of living through and during the effects of colonization is a determinant of health'. The impact of this includes historical trauma as well as contemporary racism, discrimination and stigmatization which, in turn, have negative health impacts such as increased risk for mental ill health and drug and alcohol dependency (Warwick-Booth and Cross, 2018).

Tackling the social determinants of health

The CSDH framework (Solar and Irwin, 2010: 7) proposes three broad policy approaches to tackling health inequities:

1. Targeting programmes for disadvantaged populations
2. Closing health gaps between worse-off and better-off groups
3. Addressing the social heath gradient across the whole population

The CSDH framework emphasizes that it is not enough to try to address the intermediary determinants of health; policy must also tackle the structural determinants which result in the inequitable distribution of health outcomes (Solar and Irwin, 2010). This needs to happen not just at the macro (public), meso (community) and micro (individual) levels but also at higher levels of governance, including in relation to the environment and globalization. All such strategies will need intersectoral action, social participation and empowerment. See Table 4.2 for more detail.

Woodall and Cross (2022) suggest that, in order to tackle inequalities in health, resources need to be reallocated on the basis of need – not equally, therefore, but *equitably*. The British Medical Association (2022) argues that action needs to be taken on the wider determinants of health, which have a much greater influence than healthcare services. Thus health needs to become the focus of all policy, in recognition

Table 4.2 Tackling the social determinants of health

Level	Type of policy
Globalization and environment	Policies on *stratification* to reduce inequalities and mitigate the effects of stratification
Macro level: public policies	Policies to reduce the *exposure* of disadvantaged people to health-damaging factors
Meso level: community	Policies to reduce the *vulnerabilities* of disadvantaged people
Micro level: individual interaction	Policies to reduce the *unequal consequences* of illness in social, economic and health terms

Source: Adapted from Solar and Irwin (2010: 8)

of the fact that health is influenced even before birth and is then shaped by numerous determinants across the life course: 'Policies to improve health and tackle inequalities must therefore focus on building the foundations of good mental and physical health from pre-conception through the early years and sustain these through policies that prioritise health in all sectors' (British Medical Association, 2022: 2). This focus on early years was also emphasized in Sir Michael Marmot's report, *Fair Society, Healthy Lives* (2010), as can be seen in the first of its six proposed policy objectives:

1. Give every child the best start in life
2. Enable all children, young people and adults to maximize their capabilities and have control over their lives
3. Create fair employment and good work for all
4. Ensure a healthy standard of living for all
5. Create and develop healthy and sustainable places and communities
6. Strengthen the role and impact of ill-health prevention

Marmot et al.'s *Health Equity in England: The Marmot Review 10 Years On* (2020) again emphasized the importance of the early years for tackling health inequalities. Addressing these inequalities means focusing efforts upstream: 'identifying and addressing the social determinants of health that positively or negatively affect health (e.g. lack of access to affordable nutritious food)' (Schoon and Krumwiede, 2022: 1071). Upstream issues include many things, such as unemployment, poor housing, civic unrest and lack of access to healthcare services. With reference to public understandings of health inequalities, Kane et al. argue that an ecological mindset is needed to tackle inequalities in health, but caution that the scale and complexity of the action required can lead to a 'possible sense of inevitability or disempowerment' (2022: 3). In addition to re-emphasizing the six original policy recommendations from 2010, Marmot et al. (2020) reiterate the concept of proportionate universalism: that effort should be proportional to need. In other words, efforts to enable everyone to have the most optimum health should be focused on those who are most disadvantaged in society.

Case Study 4: Fuel poverty, cold homes and health inequalities in the UK (adapted from Lee at al., 2022)

Fuel poverty and cold homes are inextricably linked. Households on low incomes facing high energy costs are more likely to experience fuel poverty, which is further exacerbated by the energy efficiency of a home. It was estimated that one in five UK households with dependent children experienced fuel poverty in 2020, and this is likely to have increased given subsequent rises in fuel costs. As of April 2023, the National Energy Action charity estimated that 7.5 million households in the UK were living in fuel poverty (Hinson et al., 2023).

Cold homes resulting from fuel poverty increase health inequalities. Living in a cold home worsens existing respiratory conditions and can also cause them. In addition, cardiovascular health, mental health and child development are also negatively impacted. In severe cases death can occur. The cost of treating people who live in fuel poverty and cold homes is significant. In 2019 it was estimated that the National Health Service spent at least £2.5 billion on treating illnesses directly related to people living in cold, damp and dangerous homes. England's excess winter deaths are higher than the northern European average. The structural determinants clearly come into play here – certain people and households are more vulnerable to fuel poverty, especially those living on low incomes, or with disabilities or chronic disease, older people, households with dependents, and minority ethnic households.

As Lee et al. point out: 'Tackling fuel poverty and health problems related to cold homes is important for reducing health inequalities in the UK. Local authorities and public health are well placed to address issues relating to fuel poverty but reducing fuel poverty also requires national action and resources. [There are] many examples of how local areas are tackling fuel poverty and reducing health inequalities, such as: targeting advice services and housing improvements, including improvements in the private rented sector; using urban regeneration to reduce fuel poverty; and partnerships between the NHS, local authorities and housing and beyond to support local populations' (2022: 5).

Summary

This chapter has described the importance of various social determinants of health in terms of their influence on health experience and health outcomes. Drawing on two models of social determinants of health has enabled us to appreciate not only the wide range of factors that impact on health but also how the interaction between these different factors is highly complex. The chapter considered issues of inequality and inequity as well as the role of structure and agency in determining health. Finally, we looked at some potential ways of tackling health inequalities. The next chapter will consider health as well-being.

Further reading

Warwick-Booth, L. (2019) *Social Inequality*. 2nd edition. London, Sage.

This text provides a comprehensive overview of social inequality as a major determinant of health. It covers key concepts and theories using a range of examples to bring the debates to life. Topics include youth and age, gender, social class, health and disability, migration, globalization, sexuality and transgender issues, and the media, among others.

5
Health as Well-being

Chapter aims

- To critically consider the idea of health as well-being
- To explore different definitions and dimensions of well-being, and how it might be experienced
- To examine how well-being might be measured

Introduction

This chapter focuses on the idea of health as well-being. It critically considers concepts of well-being and how health is related to this, starting with an exploration of different definitions of well-being. It will consider well-being in relation to Grant et al.'s (2007) three core elements of well-being – psychological, physical and social – and some other theoretical contributions, including that offered by Martin Seligman. The discussion draws on a range of research about well-being and health, using lay perspectives as a basis for the discussion. The challenges of measuring well-being are considered, taking into account how ideas about it vary according to different social factors such as culture and race/ethnicity. The chapter includes an overview of the Geneva

Charter for Well-being and ends with a brief discussion about quality of life. Before you go any further please take some time out to consider Pause for Reflection 5.1.

Pause for Reflection 5.1

What does the word 'well-being' mean to you? What kind of things does it encompass? What does well-being look like or present as? How would you describe it to someone else?

How does it relate to health? Is it the same as health or something different?

There are no right or wrong answers to these questions, but they should have caused you to begin to question what well-being is.

What is well-being?

The discussion in this chapter is closely related to the discussion in Chapter 6, which examines the idea of health as happiness. In one sense it is difficult to separate out well-being and happiness; however, even though they are intricately connected, it is possible to consider them as separate entities, and the terms are often used quite differently in research and in the wider literature. The World Health Organization, along with many countries, has been promoting a paradigm shift away from negative health outcomes such as illness and disease and towards more positive ways of viewing health in terms of well-being and happiness (Warwick-Booth and Cross, 2018).

Well-being is foregrounded in Sustainable Development Goal 3: Ensure healthy lives and promote well-being across all ages.* There is general agreement that both well-being and happiness are subjectively experienced (Woodall and Cross, 2022) and, therefore, are subjectively expressed

* See https://sustainabledevelopment.un.org/focussdgs.html.

(Hubley et al., 2021). Although we use the term well-being in common parlance (and the word is increasingly used in relation to all manner of things), it is difficult to define (Chronin de Chavez et al., 2005; Dodge et al., 2012). There is also a lack of consensus on a definition of well-being in the academic literature. However, there does appear to be some agreement that understandings and experiences of well-being concern three major domains or areas – physical, social and psychological well-being (Warwick-Booth et al., 2021).

Morrison and Bennett (2016: 416) define well-being as 'the subjective evaluation of a person's overall life'. However, as they argue, a person's subjective evaluation of their life will also reflect, in part at least, their objective material circumstances. These will include things like their relationships (or lack thereof) and their financial and employment status, as well as their physical health status. It is difficult to separate well-being from the circumstances of our everyday lives. Focusing more on the cognitive and affective aspects of well-being, Fleming and Baldwin (2020: 19) describe it as 'a positive concept with a focus on what people think and feel about their lives, such as the quality of their relationships, their positive emotions and resilience, the realisation of their potential and their overall satisfaction with life'. Well-being is generally seen as encompassing feelings as well as some kind of evaluation about satisfaction with life (Centers for Disease Control and Prevention, 2018). More broadly, Wills (2023: 4) states that well-being 'is a term widely used to describe what makes a good life'. This highlights the subjective nature of well-being and separates it from ideas about happiness.

The WHO's (1948) definition of health foregrounds well-being as follows: 'a state of complete physical, mental and social *well-being* and not merely the absence of disease or infirmity'. The use of the all-encompassing term 'well-being' in this definition has been criticized by some. For example, McDonald (2023: npn) suggests that using such a broad term is a major limitation of the definition as it means that the concept of health 'dissolves into a myriad personal subjectivities among which there is no obvious priority'. Several decades later, the WHO's (2009) definition of mental health also included the notion of well-being: 'mental health is defined as a state of well-being in which every individual realizes [their] own potential, can cope with the normal stresses of life, can work productively and fruitfully, and is able to make a contribution to [their] community'. The United Nations Declaration on the Right of Development (UN, 1986) highlights well-being in relation to development, emphasizing that the latter is (or should be) linked to the 'constant improvement of the well-being of the entire population on the basis of their active, free and meaningful participation in the development and the fair distribution of benefits'. The focus in this declaration is on populations rather than individuals.

While in western cultures well-being tends to be viewed at an individual level, in Aboriginal and Torres Strait Islander communities ideas about health include the 'social, emotional and cultural well-being of the whole community', not just individual physical well-being (Fleming et al., 2020: 19). Many Indigenous cultures view well-being in a holistic and relational way. As Williams and Mumtaz (2007: 9) state, 'mental well-being is intimately connected to emotional, physical, spiritual well-being. [Health or] well-being is synonymous with self-determination and is generally much more a collective phenomenon within which the individual is metaphysically indistinct from their extended family, ancestors, land and historical tribal context.' In contrast, in the context of westernized and capitalist democracies, experiences of well-being are often infused with imperial power dynamics that 'structure everyday contexts and the internalized realities of those who inhabit them' (Williams and Mumtaz, 2007: 11).

This highlights the socially constructed nature of well-being and the fact that subjective experiences of well-being are influenced (and constrained) by many different factors. Thus, well-being might mean one thing to one person and a very different thing to someone else. Our ideas about well-being will also likely change across different situations and across our lifespan. Grant et al. (2007) used the WHO's definition of health as a starting point for thinking about how to conceptualize well-being. Drawing on psychological, philosophical and sociological definitions of well-being in the wider literature, they conceived it as having three distinct aspects: psychological, physical and social (see Box 5.1).

Box 5.1: Core elements of well-being (adapted from Grant et al., 2007: 52 and Cross, 2020: 62)

Psychological: concerned with the ability to cope or adapt to circumstances; includes agency, satisfaction, self-respect and capabilities

Physical: concerned with healthy functioning, fitness and performance; includes nourishment, shelter, clothing, healthcare and mobility

Social: concerned with the quality of interpersonal relationships and community involvement; includes participating in community, being accepted in public, and helping others

---

Like Grant et al. (2007), Laverack (2004) separates well-being into three different types: physical (concerned with healthy functioning, fitness and physical capacity), social (concerned with interpersonal relationships and community involvement) and mental (concerned with the ability to cope and things like self-esteem). According to Johnson et al. (2016) well-being has different elements, including having our basic psychological needs met, experiencing positive emotions, engaging with others, having meaningful relationships and accomplishing our goals. This brings in the importance of social well-being and having a sense of purpose or meaning in life. Gu et al. (2015) point out that well-being is often closely associated with mental health. In addition, people like White (2017) have highlighted the importance of the natural environment for well-being, particularly for rural communities in low- and middle-income countries. In the face of significant environmental degradation, we are seeing an increasing general recognition that well-being (and health) and our physical world are intimately connected. This will be discussed in more detail in Chapter 8.

As can be appreciated from the discussion so far, notions of well-being can be categorized, broadly speaking, in two main ways: firstly, as hedonic or subjective well-being, and, secondly, as eudaimonic or social well-being. The first is concerned with intrinsic factors such as how people feel and what they think (Das et al., 2020); the second is concerned with how extrinsic factors, such as relationships and the external environment, affect people's well-being (Phongsavan et al., 2006).

Theories of well-being

Early research on lay ideas about health identified 'a general sense of well-being' as one of three main responses to the question 'what does being healthy mean?' (along with physical fitness and the absence of symptoms of disease) (Bauman, cited in Morrison and Bennett, 2016: 12). Canadian epidemiologist Ronald Labonté's (1998) model of health places well-being at the heart of it. As you can see from Figure 5.1, Labonté conceives of health as having three dimensions – physical, mental and social (these dimensions, and others,

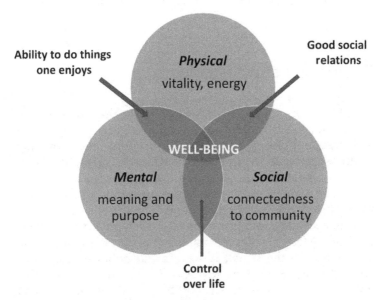

Figure 5.1: Labonté's model of health
Source: Adapted from Orme et al. (2003: 287)

were discussed in detail in Chapter 2). Labonté places well-being in the centre of the model where these three dimensions overlap with one another in a Venn diagram formation. For Labonté all three dimensions of health are crucial to well-being.

Psychologist Martin Seligman's (2011) theory of subjective well-being has five subjective elements: positive emotion, engagement, relationships, meaning and accomplishment (abbreviated as PERMA). Seligman (2018: 334) suggests that PERMA is 'a theory of the building blocks of well-being'. This theory reflects how people feel as well as how they function (Forgeard et al., 2011). Each component can be measured independently even though they are all (inter)related. Whilst PERMA has been used in many ways, Seligman (2018) acknowledges that the pursuit of a sufficient theory of well-being is a continuing endeavour. In response to an increased interest in well-being, the What Works Centre for Wellbeing (UK) was set up in 2015. The main purpose of the centre is to understand and collate evidence on how to improve well-being, with a view to driving the inclusion of a well-being agenda in public policy (Bache, 2019).*

Experiences of well-being

In addition to objective measures of health such as life expectancy and healthy life years, subjective well-being is increasingly being viewed as crucial to understanding health experience (Morrison and Bennett, 2016). Research by Angner et al. (2009) found that, for older people, subjective well-being was a better predictor of happiness than objective measures of physical health such as illness. For many Indigenous communities (such as First Nations, Inuit and Métis peoples in Canada) experiences of well-being are shaped by the social, economic and political legacies of colonization, as well as diversity (Williams and Mumtaz, 2007). Wills (2023) points out that more egalitarian and

* See https://whatworkswellbeing.org for more information.

community-oriented societies report higher levels of well-being. Ideas about well-being vary according to different social factors, such as culture, race/ethnicity, gender and education level, as well as access to material support. Many studies also link well-being to income levels (Warwick-Booth and Cross, 2018).

As stated previously, for many people well-being is primarily concerned with mental health rather than other dimensions of health, such that mental health and well-being become synonymous with one another. For example, research by Hallam et al. (2018) explored the benefits of physical activity on mental health and well-being and conflated the two throughout the study. Some research has pointed to the importance of green and blue spaces for promoting experiences of well-being (see Box 5.2).

The Body Positivity movement promotes the idea of health and well-being at any body size, challenging 'status quo beauty ideals by portraying and promoting diverse physical appearances' (Stevens and Griffiths, 2020: 181). Social media platforms have enabled such messages to proliferate, with research on this showing a clear link between higher body satisfaction (at any size) and a positive body image, and improved emotional and psychological well-being (Nelson et al., 2022; O'Hara et al., 2021). Conversely (and perhaps not surprisingly) weight-related stigma leads to poor well-being (O'Hara et al., 2021). Please take some time to consider Pause for Reflection 5.2 before reading any further.

Pause for Reflection 5.2

Well-being is a multifaceted concept. Take some time to think about how you would measure it. How might you find out if someone has positive well-being (or not)? Would you use subjective measures (such as asking them how they feel) or objective measures (such as monitoring physical body (re)actions)? Or perhaps a combination of both?

Box 5.2: Places, spaces and social relations (from Bagnall, 2023)

A 2023 global review by the UK-based What Works Centre for Wellbeing explored the impact of changes in community infrastructure on people's well-being. The review found there was 'strong evidence that community hubs and community development improve social relations, individual and community wellbeing and that different types of interventions can have impacts on different aspects of wellbeing ... For example:

- Changes to green and blue spaces, such as parks and canal paths, predominantly affect individual well-being, especially physical activity and mental well-being
- Changes to community hubs, and community development, bring about positive changes in social connections, skills and knowledge, and social cohesion
- Events such as festivals, street parties, and other short-term changes in how community spaces are used bring about positive changes in hedonic well-being (also known as fun!), social connections and a sense of belonging and identity'

However, the review also found that these positive impacts were not universal. For example, community events can sometimes lead to some people feeling excluded.

Measuring well-being

The relatively recent focus on well-being has led to questions about how it can and should be measured (Dodge et al., 2012). Many people, such as psychologists Forgeard and colleagues (2011), for example, question the value of gross domestic product (GDP) as a measure of a country's success or progress. Indeed, in 1968, Bobby Kennedy famously said that GDP 'measures everything except that which is worthwhile' (cited in British Medical Association, 2022: 14). Whilst GDP is easy to track and measure, it is a rather limited way of establishing what constitutes success. In addition, as Forgeard et al. (2011: 80) note, 'the GDP of a nation increases with each sale of antidepressant medication, with each divorce pronounced, and with each prison built', none of which would be equated with any sense of well-being. Hubley et al. (2021) point out that many of the epidemiological measures used to evaluate health are physical and therefore reinforce the dominance of medical, biological ideas about what health is. Ilona Kickbusch (2012), well known for her influence on health promotion and global health, argues that success in health must be measured in different ways. She maintains that it is not sufficient to focus solely on economic production and outputs. Rather, well-being and quality of life should be taken into account. Like others, Kickbusch (2012) argues that it is no longer enough to measure success or progress by simply using economic indicators such as GDP. Many governments have now introduced measures of well-being and quality of life in order to obtain indicators of progress above and beyond material and economic ones (Cross et al., 2021b). Rather than relying simply on GDP as a measure of success, some governments are now more interested in subjective experiences of health and well-being. For example, Canada has a comprehensive Index of Well-Being that has eight domains:

1. Living standard
2. Health
3. Environment
4. Democratic engagement
5. Time use
6. Education
7. Community vitality
8. Leisure and culture*

In 2018 the Well-being Economy Government network was formed to 'transform economic systems so that they deliver collective well-being' (British Medical Association, 2022: 16). The network includes Iceland, New Zealand, Scotland, Wales

---

* For further information see https://uwaterloo.ca/canadian-index-wellbeing.

and Finland. In 2019, New Zealand published a Well-being Budget that outlined five government well-being priorities: improving mental health, reducing child poverty, addressing the inequalities faced by Indigenous Māori and Pacific Island people, thriving in a digital age, and transitioning to a low-emission, sustainable economy.* In the UK there have been more recent proposals to measure well-being 'alongside more traditional economic measures' (British Medical Association, 2022: 2). The BMA's 2022 report recognizes that well-being is an economic and social asset, crucial for growth and national prosperity. England's Office of National Statistics Health Index has ten domains, including one specific to subjective well-being, and in 2015 Wales published the Well-being of Future Generations Act, which details seven well-being goals for the country as follows:

1. A prosperous Wales
2. A resilient Wales
3. A healthier Wales
4. A more equal Wales
5. A Wales of more cohesive communities
6. A Wales of vibrant culture and thriving Welsh language
7. A globally responsible Wales

The purpose of the Act is promote sustainable decision-making to ensure future generations have at least the same quality of life as the current one, and its goals encompass social, economic, environmental and cultural well-being.†

As stated in previous chapters, the concept of well-being is central to many Indigenous communities' perspectives on health, which incorporate ideas about the (inter)relationships of all things living and past, including the physical world. However, a lot of the research on well-being is dominated by 'western' ideology, which then informs how subjective understandings and experiences are investigated or determined. Tremblay and Martin (2023: 105) advocate for Etuaptmumk

---

* See   https://www.treasury.govt.nz/publications/wellbeing-budget/well being-budget-2021-securing-our-recovery for further details.
† For more information see https://www.gov.wales/well-being-of-future -generations-wales.

or Two-Eyed Seeing as 'a guiding principle that fosters the respectful and equitable consideration of Indigenous and Western ways of knowing and understanding'. They go on to argue that 'using both or many diverse views or eyes creates a unique and alternative vision that values the contributions of [both] ways of knowing'.

Research on subjective well-being tends to ask people questions about how satisfied they are with their lives, how they feel and whether or not they consider that life is worthwhile (World Economic Forum, 2015). One of the criticisms of subjective well-being measures is that the indicators used to assess levels of well-being often reflect the values of those who have designed the means of investigation and not necessarily the values of those participating in the research (Forgeard et al., 2011). However, a salient point perhaps is that, whatever way well-being is measured, it tends to rely on a person's own judgement of their well-being rather than that imposed on them by other people. This leaves people free to decide what well-being means to them and respond accordingly. Interestingly, in their research into body positivity and well-being, Vendemia and Robinson (2022) asked participants to rate themselves on three qualities of subjective well-being: happiness, success and life satisfaction.

Since the concept of well-being is so complex and subjective, Forgeard et al. (2011) have recommended what they call a 'dashboard' approach, proposing that well-being be measured in lots of different ways to reflect both objective and subjective elements. Kickbusch (2012), in agreement with Forgeard et al. (2011), reports on the French government's 2008 Commission on the Measurement of Economic Performance and Social Progress, which recommended that 'the time is ripe for our measurement system to shift emphasis from measuring economic production to measuring people's well-being. And measures of well-being should be put in a context of sustainability'. It also noted how 'well-being is multidimensional and that its various dimensions should be considered simultaneously: material living standard (income, consumption and wealth); health; education, personal activities including work, political voice and governance; social connections and relationships; environment (present and future conditions); and insecurity, of an economic as well as a physical nature' (Kickbusch, 2012: 6).

> **Box 5.3: Measuring well-being – the Warwick-Edinburgh Mental Well-being Scale**
>
> The Warwick-Edinburgh Mental Well-being Scale (WEMWBS) (Tennant et al., 2007) is comprised of fourteen items that have to be responded to using a five-point scale: from 1 which indicates *none of the time*, through to five which indicates *all of the time*. It is a measure of subjective well-being in which the items (statements) are framed in a positive way. People complete the scale and end up with a single score.

Some measures of well-being have been criticized for focusing too much on the individual and not taking into account external factors that might impact on subjective well-being, such as climate change and the sociopolitical context (Cross et al., 2021b). The Warwick-Edinburgh Mental Well-being Scale (see Box 5.3) is a good example of this. Further critiques note that the focus on the individual in these kinds of measures means that they often fail to take community well-being into account, even though it is inextricably linked to individual well-being (Atkinson et al., 2019). In support of this, White (2017) argues that *relational* well-being is more important than individual well-being, particularly in more collectivist societies (such as Bangladesh and Zambia) where a higher value is placed on community. In such contexts, White contends, relational well-being is more important than individual well-being since it is crucial for social inclusion and societal change. The research on well-being also tends to be dominated by the global north, which leads to concerns about the generalizability of findings and the lack of attention to the cultural, environmental and historical differences between the global north and the global south (Beida et al., 2017). In addition, well-being measures have been criticized for being deductionist and individualist constructs that distract from the structural factors that impact on health. Finally it is argued that some researchers have conflated well-being with other things such as 'happiness, quality of life or life satisfaction', have tended to ignore the fact that well-being is more complex and 'multifaceted', and have, at times, confined it to 'one construct (often life satisfaction)' (Forgeard et al., 2011: 81).

The Geneva Charter for Well-being

The tenth global conference on health promotion, held in Geneva, Switzerland and online in December 2021, resulted in the publication of the Geneva Charter for Well-being. Each of the previous nine conferences had resulted in some sort of charter or statement, but this was the first one to put well-being front and centre in the title of the resulting publication and throughout it. For details of the Geneva Charter for Well-being see Box 5.4.

Box 5.4: From the Geneva Charter for Well-being (WHO, 2021)

Foundations of well-being
Well-being societies provide the foundations for all members of current and future generations to thrive on a healthy planet, no matter where they live. Such societies apply bold policies and transformative approaches that are underpinned by:

- A positive vision of health that integrates physical, mental, spiritual and social well-being.
- The principles of human rights, social and environmental justice, solidarity, gender and inter-generational equity, and peace.
- A commitment to sustainable low-carbon development grounded in reciprocity and respect among humans and making peace with Nature.
- New indicators of success, beyond GDP, that take account of human and planetary well-being and lead to new priorities for public spending.
- The focus of health promotion on empowerment, inclusivity, equity, and meaningful participation.

21st century health promotion response
Creating well-being societies requires coordinated action in five areas:

1. Value, respect and nurture planet Earth and its ecosystems
2. Design an equitable economy that serves human development within planetary and local ecological boundaries
3. Develop healthy public policy for the common good
4. Achieve universal health coverage
5. Address the impacts of digital transformation

Stewarding a flourishing future
Well-being is a political choice. ... [It] requires a whole-of-society approach involving action across all levels, stakeholders and sectors, from communities and within organizations to regional and national government. The role of health promotion is to catalyse and support this movement by:

- Ensuring that people and communities are enabled to take control of their health and lead fulfilling lives with a sense of meaning and purpose, in harmony with nature, through education, culturally relevant health literacy, meaningful empowerment and engagement.
- Enabling, mediating and advocating for a unifying approach to creating well-being societies by shaping the determinants of health in all settings.
- Ensuring that promotive, preventive, curative, rehabilitative and palliative health and social services are of high quality, affordable, accessible and acceptable and are provided according to needs, especially for those often left behind.

Source: https://www.who.int/publications/m/item/the-geneva-charter-for-well-being

As noted previously in this chapter, the WHO included well-being in its seminal definition of health; however, the 2021 global conference in Geneva was the first conference to foreground well-being in its resulting output. The conference charter, accessible in full on the WHO website, covers a lot of ground in outlining what is required to build a more sustainable future for everyone's well-being. It nicely demonstrates what has been discussed in this chapter: that 'well-being is best understood as a multifaceted phenomenon that can be assessed by measuring a wide array of subjective and objective constructs' (Forgeard et al., 2011: 79). Put simply, well-being is related to what it means to have a 'good' life. It is strongly associated with what it means to be human and to live well (Atkinson et al., 2019). In the last section of this chapter we will briefly consider the concept of quality of life in its connection to well-being.

Quality of life

The concept of quality of life is another important factor for well-being (Cross et al., 2021a). Like well-being, it is a subjectively experienced, value-laden phenomenon which is, therefore, socially constructed (Green et al., 2019). However, most people would agree that quality of life is important, even more so than the number of years lived (Woodall and Cross, 2021). Despite the widespread use of the term, there is no agreed definition of 'quality of life'. In fact, it is defined in different ways in the literature, with a general appreciation that it encompasses many social, environmental, psychological and physical values (Theofilou, 2013). This is supported by research demonstrating how quality of life is affected by many factors. For example, Ward et al. (2019) show that, for older people in Ireland, quality of life is not just about physical health and ageing but also concerned with things like loneliness and social participation. As Theofilou (2013: 151) notes: 'The concept of quality of life broadly encompasses how an individual measures the "goodness" of multiple aspects of their life.' Like well-being, quality of life is understood to have subjective and objective elements and the concept has been introduced to better appreciate human experience beyond comparably simplistic measures such as rates of deaths and disease (Karimi and Brazier, 2016).

Case Study 5: Hygge and fika – Scandinavian well-being practices

Hygge (Denmark)
Hygge is a Danish word that, according to the Cambridge Dictionary, refers to a sense of warmth, being at ease or comfortable, and feeling safe and cosy. In recent years, Hygge has become associated with ideas about well-being more generally. Colino and Young (2022: npn) state that 'practicing hygge is about doing things we know are good for lowering stress and boosting wellness, from drinking warm soothing beverages to spending time with people we care about'. But hygge is also about simple pleasures such as lighting candles, baking and being with others. Neilsen and Ma (2021) note how Denmark is often ranked as one of the world's happiest countries, suggesting that there may be a link between the practice of hygge and this consistent outcome. The social aspect of hygge is important, highlighting the integral nature of personal and collective well-being.

Fika (Sweden)
Fika is the Swedish cultural practice of slowing down and taking a break, typically to have a cup of coffee and chat to someone, maybe over a piece of cake or some other treat (Caprioli et al., 2021). The social nature of this is important as it is as much about having an opportunity to connect with others as it is about having a break for a hot drink or a snack.

Hygge and fika are traditional Scandinavian practices embedded in the cultures and habits of Danish and Swedish people; both enhance subjective and collective well-being. It is claimed by some that these practices have been oversimplified and superficially promoted in other cultural contexts such that their complexity and meaning have been lost (Caproli et al., 2021). However, for many, the central appeal of both practices is their promotion of social cohesion – spending quality time with other people (Cassinger et al., 2019). This is, of course, an important component of well-being.

Summary

This chapter has explored the concept of well-being in relation to health. Like health, well-being is understood and experienced in different ways. It is a complex and multi-faceted idea that is influenced by several different factors. The chapter has highlighted the socially constructed nature of well-being and how it is context-dependent. Finally, we have explored the complexities of measuring well-being. However, as noted, well-being is now receiving increasing attention as a measure of success.

Further reading

For further detail about happiness and health see Bache, I. (2019) How does evidence matter? Understanding 'what works' for well-being. *Social Indicators Research,* 142, 1153–73.

Author's summary: 'In 2015 the UK launched an independent What Works Centre for Wellbeing, co-funded by government departments and various agencies, which aims to develop a "strong and credible evidence base" to help promote well-being in policy. Yet while there is widespread agreement that evidence matters in policy-making, it is far from clear what kind of evidence matters, in what circumstances and to what extent. In this context, this article presents the findings of research exploring with policy-makers and stakeholders issues in the use of evidence in relation to well-being in public policy. In particular, it highlights evidence as a specific form of (research-based) knowledge and considers the importance of this relative to other forms of knowledge: political, professional and experiential. This approach highlights a broader understanding of 'what works' beyond the relatively technical sense often employed to describe the work of the What Works Centre and in the use of evidence more generally.'

See also: whatworkswellbeing.org

6
Health as Happiness

Chapter aims

- To critically consider the idea of health as happiness
- To explore different definitions and dimensions of happiness, and how it might be experienced
- To examine how happiness might be measured

Introduction

In the past two decades happiness has become more generally linked to health and health experience in the broader literature. Some people would even argue that to be happy is to be healthy. Happiness indices now offer a way of measuring quality of life outside of economic means. This chapter will explore what happiness *is* and how it relates to concepts of what it means to be healthy. Happiness is considered firstly at the individual level and then at societal level. Happiness research is drawn upon throughout the chapter to make sense of what health as happiness is about. Reference is made to relevant theoretical constructs of happiness. There will also be some discussion of how happiness can be measured and achieved, drawing on narratives of health and happiness from the wider literature. The chapter concludes with a case study about happiness, health and social media.

What is happiness?

There has been increased attention paid to happiness in the research on health in the past few decades (Fortier and Morgan, 2022), coupled with a broader move towards positive psychology, which has become a recognized (and popular) sub-discipline (Steptoe, 2019). As noted in the previous chapter, 'the WHO and many countries are experiencing what can be described as a paradigm shift, with a move away from concerns about illness and specific diseases and more of a focus on well-being and happiness' (Warwick-Booth and Cross, 2018: 25). This shift is reflected in many areas. Chapter 5 focused on the idea of health as well-being. Like well-being, happiness is fundamentally linked to health (Woodall and Cross, 2022). Some people conceptualize happiness as part of subjective well-being (Forgeard et al., 2011) or even both as being one and the same thing (Steptoe, 2019). For others happiness and health are the same thing – feeling happy is feeling healthy and vice versa (Cloninger and Zohar, 2011). In some studies happiness is simply about subjective experience (Guerci et al., 2022). As Fortier and Morgan (2022: 8560) state, 'while there is a conceptual overlap between happiness, well-being, quality of life, mental health, and life satisfaction, a growing number of studies are showing that happiness is different/unique'. Well-being and happiness are often conflated but, for the purposes of this book, we are considering them as separate concepts.

Happiness, much like well-being, is arguably another highly subjective phenomenon. What makes one person happy will not necessarily make another person feel the same way. But what is happiness? There does seem to be some consistency across different cultures about how happiness is defined (e.g. in terms of inner harmony, or balance and connectedness with other people) (Delle Fave et al., 2016), but there is a general lack of a universal meaning (Diener et al., 2017). Woodall and Cross (2022) observe that happiness is simply a human experience that is the opposite of sadness. However, many people argue that it is more than that. It is generally agreed that happiness is a multifaceted phenomenon which is experienced and conceptualized differently by different people (Krys et al., 2021). Elsewhere in the literature, happiness is seen as a component of well-being alongside many others (for example, life satisfaction or positive relationships) (Guerci et al., 2022). The importance that people place on happiness varies considerably and is tied up with ideological and cultural values. As shown in research by Wathne (2014), for example, for some people being fat brings a feeling of happiness. This is inextricably bound up with socially constructed meanings of fatness, which is seen as being of value in some contexts rather than problematic or simply bad for health. In India the notion of happiness is fundamentally bound up with ancient philosophy expressed through the practice of Yoga and in ancient documents such as Sanskrit texts (Bhattacharyya et al., 2019).

Happiness is often conceived of as pleasure or hedonic experience, which tends to be related to a transient and temporary state. Interestingly, happiness is also described by some as an 'attitude' (Miething et al., 2020). Philosopher John Rawls (cited in Forgeard et al., 2011: 93) conceived of happiness as having two parts: 'the successful execution of a rational life plan, and that individual's state of mind'. This is an individualistic perspective on happiness, focused at the personal level. Another individualistic definition is offered by Schueller and Seligman (cited in Fortier and Morgan, 2022: 8559): 'happiness has been theorized as the holistic experience of pleasure, engagement, and meaningfulness'. See Box 6.1 for an example of a further definition of this type.

Box 6.1: A definition of happiness (Lyubomirsky, cited in Daniel-González et al., 2023: 955)

'Happiness is a feeling of joy, satisfaction, and living in a state of well-being which, at the same time, leads people to feel that they have a meaningful life worth living.'

There is, then, a dominant idea that happiness is subjective and individually located. However, this is not the only way of thinking about happiness. Daniel-González et al. (2023) note how happiness is culturally located, arguing that concepts and meanings of happiness vary across cultures and also change over time. As Jo et al. (2020: 921) point out, ideas about happiness are shaped by normative beliefs as well as by culture. By way of example, they point out how happiness is 'relatively self-oriented in the US', while in Eastern cultures it is pursued through 'social engagement' and experienced by spending time with other people (family and friends).

The concept of interdependent happiness has been introduced into the literature subsequent to the dominance of life satisfaction as a happiness indicator. Interdependent happiness refers to a 'more relationship-oriented view of happiness – emphasizing harmony with others, quiescence, and ordinariness' (Krys et al., 2021: 2199). It is generally associated with more collectivist societies and is fundamentally linked to social health. Collectivist societies are those where greater priority is given to community rather than the individual. Generally, 'non-western' countries tend more towards collectivism than individualism as compared with 'western' countries. Krys et al. (2021) acknowledge that there is some overlap between interdependent happiness and life satisfaction, but argue that the former is more associated with the quality of our relationships whilst the latter is more associated with personal achievements. Interdependent happiness is also arguably associated with the concept of social capital. Research carried out in Japan found a positive relationship between happiness and social capital with respect to the following components of the latter: trust, social connections/interactions and social participation (Tsuruta et al., 2019). Such findings highlight the importance of collectivism for subjective happiness and the crucial role that other people play in our experiences of happiness (for better or for worse). Tsuruta et al. (2019: 251) concluded that 'the relationship between social capital and health in terms of happiness is important in creating a lively society in which citizens support one another, in addition to promoting physical and mental well-being'.

We also often talk about the pursuit of happiness, or happiness as a state of being. Beida et al. (2017) note how happiness is strongly and independently related to mental health (alongside other things such as optimism, life satisfaction and resilience). We also refer to happiness as a feeling (affect, emotion), although some people caution that we should not confuse happiness with cheerfulness, which can be conceptualized as either a mood state or a personality trait (Ruch, 2014). The Happiness Research Institute (2020) proposes that happiness has three dimensions:

1. Cognitive (i.e. life satisfaction)
2. Affective (i.e. positive and negative affect)
3. Eudemonic (i.e. life purpose)

Professor of psychology and epidemiology Andrew Steptoe (2019: 339) reinforces this idea in his paper on health and happiness as follows: 'happiness encompasses several constructs, including affective well-being (feelings of joy and pleasure), eudemonic well-being (sense of meaning and purpose in life), and evaluative well-being (life-satisfaction)'. The parallels between these two ways of conceptualizing happiness can clearly be seen; however, as stated previously, a final, agreed-upon definition still eludes us. Consequently, Hofmann (2019: 95) contends that we need to 'harness' happiness given the vagueness of the term, while Fortier and Morgan (2022) argue that more work is needed to clarify and define what happiness actually is.

Happiness and health

Despite the definitional challenges outlined in the previous section there is strong empirical evidence that happiness and health are related and interact with one another. As argued by Wang et al. (2022) much of the attention paid to happiness and health in the broader literature is predicated on the assumption that interventions might be implemented that could make people happier and, therefore, healthier. This has been a particular focus of public policy in many countries in the past two decades, and, of course, it makes sense. If we can find the key to creating and sustaining happiness, then health should follow suit. The main question, however, is: are happier people healthier, or are healthier people happier? As stated previously, several factors contribute to happiness, some of which will be discussed in more detail later in this chapter. These include income, employment and relationship status. For example, an Indonesian study using data from the Indonesian Family Life Survey found that 'happier Indonesians earned more money, were more likely to be married, were less likely to be divorced or unemployed, and were in better health' (Sujarwoto, 2021: 679), whilst Jo et al.'s (2020) research into happiness in the Korean context found a positive relationship between happiness and economic status and educational levels.

Happiness is a good predictor of associated constructs such as life satisfaction and positive mental health (Fortier and Morgan, 2022). 'Happy individuals are less likely to report adverse mental health' (Burns and Crisp, 2021: 375). Happiness is considered to be a 'buffer' or protective mechanism for poorer health experience. Many studies show that higher levels of self-reported health are associated with higher levels of self-reported happiness (Liu et al., 2021). Wang et al.'s (2022) research in China found that happier people rated their health better than their unhappier counterparts. This was generally irrespective of socioeconomic factors, relationships, age and so on. Happy people are more likely to be optimistic, have better coping skills and are more resilient to adversity (Evli and Şimşek, 2022). All of these factors are also closely related to better mental health. In addition, there is a great deal of empirical evidence showing a positive relationship between happiness and all-cause mortality: the higher the level of happiness, the lower the likelihood of premature death (Steptoe, 2019). This pattern appears to be consistent across different countries.

Happiness is also strongly associated with objective measures of health such as living longer, suffering less ill health and reporting better levels of subjective health experience. As a result, happiness is emerging as a key aspiration for many societies (Wang et al., 2022). Gyasi et al. (2023: 113) note how the concept of happiness 'incorporates feelings of satisfying engagement with social and physical environments'. Clark et al. (2017) report that social connections have a large part to play in people's subjective experiences of happiness, which highlights the importance of the social dimension of health. Research by Lawrence et al. (2019) on marriage, health and happiness found that people who reported being happily married were twice as likely to report being in better health than those who were unhappily married; the latter also had a nearly 40 per cent greater likelihood of dying over the follow-up period of the study. In addition, the researchers found that general happiness was associated with increased likelihood of reporting being happily married and with better self-reported health.

Fortier and Morgan (2022) observed how happiness is influenced by the interaction between physical activity and optimism, although they also mention that this interaction is mediated by two other things – physical health and social functioning. Interestingly, however, happiness does appear to be associated with the adoption of healthier behaviours (Trudel-Fitzgerald et al., 2019). The happier someone reports themselves to be, the more likely they are to engage in behaviours that are better for their health. However, health psychologist Kate Tapper (2021) cautions against pursuing health at the expense of happiness, noting that many things which are deemed 'unhealthy' actually bring a lot of pleasure, and that the pursuit of health for its own sake might either reduce happiness or leave little time to cultivate it.

Before you move on to the next section please take some time to carry out Pause for Reflection 6.1.

Pause for Reflection 6.1

Take some time to reflect on what makes you happy or, conversely, what makes you unhappy. Try to create a list and see if you can group different factors together under some subheadings. You might also want to talk to other people about this and find out what makes them happy. No doubt you will find that there are some common themes but that everyone has a personal perspective on this.

Determinants of happiness

Happiness is determined and influenced by different things. Steptoe (2019) acknowledges that many factors will impact on happiness, including genetics, personality, education, marital status, family, socioeconomic status, stress exposure, time use and activities, and social network. This is not an exhaustive list, however, and you may have come up with some ideas in Pause for Reflection 6.1 that are not reflected in Steptoe's account. For example, our physical environment may impact on our happiness: think of being too cold, or too hot, or having noisy disruptive neighbours. Our homes matter too. In research conducted in Iran, Javani et al. (2019) found a relationship between the amount of daylight experienced by women in their homes and their levels of happiness. The authors concluded that people who 'spend the majority of their time indoors (e.g. housewives, children, elderly individuals, and people with disability) are most dependent on architecture and environmental designs for their well-being, and therefore are more affected by design decisions' (Javani et al., 2019: 103).

It is not just our homes that influence happiness, but outdoor spaces too. Buckley has written about the benefit of outdoor spaces for mental and emotional health. He carried out a study to try to determine whether 'people are happy because they visit parks, or do they visit parks because they are happy?' (Buckley 2020: 1410). The majority of the respondents (82 per cent) said that they were happy because they visited parks. In addition, 87.5 per cent said that they felt short-term emotional benefits from doing so ('feeling happier or generally more positive'), 60 per cent that they had experienced medium-term relief from stress ('feeling regenerated, more relaxed, recovered from stress'), and 20 per cent that they had experienced long-term changes in their worldview ('feeling greater clarity, or purpose, or meaning in one's life, able to see what is important'). Buckley notes that people who do not visit parks tend to be, on average, less happy or healthy than those who do. Of course, there could be any number of reasons for this; however, the positive impact of engaging with, and spending time in, green and blue spaces has been demonstrated many times, whether in terms of well-being, mental health, happiness or health in general. But access to such outside spaces is not always a positive experience on every level. Research carried out in China by Liu et al. (2021) with nearly 12,000 people across twenty-eight provinces showed that happiness was affected by air pollution. Poor air quality is an increasing concern in many countries and has negative impacts on health and longevity. Generally, people's subjective happiness is lower when there is more air pollution. Liu et al. (2021: npn) found that 'air pollution has significant negative effects on residents' happiness'. This finding is consistent with research done in other countries, such as Taiwan, where air pollution was found to have a negative impact on young people's happiness (Lin et al., 2019), and Pakistan, where Rafique et al. (2022) found that air pollution had a significantly negative impact on people's happiness.

Research involving Korean rural populations showed that levels of happiness were 'correlated with age, income, violence, social support, subjective health, depression, and suicidal ideation' (Jo et al., 2020: 915). Older adults (aged 60 and above) reported higher levels of happiness than adolescents (aged 15–19), and happiness was affected by social support (or lack of it). At a personal level, an intolerance of uncertainty negatively affects a person's happiness (Evli and Şimşek, 2022). In a Turkish study involving adolescent participants, Evli and Şimşek (2022) found that the COVID-19 pandemic had a negative impact on happiness. Personality traits can play a part too. Optimism is often associated with individual disposition (Fortier and Morgan, 2022), and is linked to happiness as it relates to expectations of positive outcomes (Steptoe, 2019). Research carried out in Mexico with medical students found that higher levels of happiness were predicted by higher levels of self-esteem, resilience and social support (Daniel-González et al., 2023). The authors concluded that self-esteem and resilience were important, at an individual level, for realizing happiness. Other research has also shown that self-esteem is a major psychological resource for greater happiness (Guerci et al., 2022).

Many things might bring personal happiness and, as has been pointed out, these will vary from person to person depending on what they value. For some people, material possessions, wealth, professional success and status are important to happiness. For example, as noted above, Jo et al.'s (2020) research in the Korean context found a positive relationship between happiness and economic status and educational levels. However, in wealthier societies increases in wealth are not associated with increases in happiness (Layard, 2011). Greater inequality leads to greater unhappiness. Economist Richard Layard (2011: 4) therefore argued that 'the time is ready for radical cultural change, away from a culture of selfishness and materialism, which fails to satisfy, towards one where we care more for each other's happiness – and make that the guiding raison d'être for our lives'. Research from urban China on happiness and housing wealth is indicative of this, showing that owning one house increases happiness, but owning more than one has diminishing returns (Cheng et al., 2020). More importantly, inequality in housing wealth seems to be more significant for happiness. Where people see others like them with more housing wealth, and feel that is unattainable, there is greater unhappiness. Cheng et al. (2020) refer to this as a 'jealousy effect'. It appears that making relative comparisons with others who have more housing wealth is the cause of unhappiness, but the actual cause of that cause is inequality. A substantial amount of research has shown that the average happiness of a country's population does not correlate well with average income. In addition, a rise in GDP does not necessarily result in a rise in reported happiness; in fact, an opposite effect has been observed in some cases – happiness scores have actually decreased, particularly for people on the lowest incomes (Tomlinson and Kelly, 2013).

As briefly mentioned earlier, social support and relationships with other people are key factors for happiness. For some, happiness comes from the quality of their relationships with significant others rather than from wealth or status. Research consistently shows that social support plays a significant role in the promotion of individual happiness in older people (Moeini et al., 2019). Ramos et al.'s (2022) study appears to show that a functional and supportive family environment during childhood and adolescence provides a basis for good family relationships in adulthood, and that this is then associated with better health and happiness. Relationships are important for health. A substantial amount of evidence points to the value of marriage for health, as compared with being divorced, separated, never married or widowed (Lawrence et al., 2019), although the benefits of this tend to be greater for men than for women. Conversely, an unhappy marriage is bad for health. The causal relationships between marriage, happiness and health are, however, complex, and Lawrence et al. (2019: 1541) note that 'general happiness may be particularly important in the relationship between marital happiness, marital status, and health'. Research on health and happiness in Australia, the United States, Britain and Indonesia by Clark et al. (2017) found that the quality of people's social relationships and their mental and physical health impacted on their subjective experiences of happiness more than their social economic status did. Similarly, a study carried out by the London School of Economics (LSE, 2016) found that human misery was connected more closely with failed relationships and poor mental and physical health than with economic circumstances.

Physical activity is also a determinant of happiness. Research shows that engaging in physical activity even in small doses (e.g. one day a week) significantly promotes happiness; this includes activities such as gardening and active transport (walking or cycling), which are also positively linked to happiness (Fortier and Morgan, 2022). In terms of greatest return, engaging in short physical activity sessions just a few days a week seems to be the best strategy for improving happiness (Fortier and Morgan, 2022). This appears to be a cross-cultural phenomenon; for example, research among older people in Ghana showed that physical inactivity was significantly related to lower levels of happiness (Gyasi et al., 2023).

Buettner et al. (2020) carried out a study involving experts in empirical happiness research to explore what they thought was the means to greater happiness. See Box 6.2 for the resulting recommendations. It should be noted, however, that all of the people involved in this study were from the global north, and therefore, it could be assumed, shared a similar set of ideological values.

Box 6.2: Ways to greater happiness (Buettner et al., 2020)

Individual strategies:

- Connect with other people
- Seek meaning
- Be active
- Cultivate a positive outlook
- Care for one's health
- Find a way of life that suits you
- Keep learning

Policy strategies:

- Invest in happiness research
- Invest in good governance
- Support vulnerable people
- Improve the social climate (in particular by promoting voluntary work and supporting non-profits)
- Invest in healthcare
- Invest in education
- Support work (through improvement in working conditions and reducing employment)
- Focus on economic stability
- Introduce higher tax rates (in order to support all of the above policy recommendations)

As has been demonstrated, the relationship between health and happiness is a complex one. A final point worth noting is that feelings of happiness can also result from our biochemistry. Although this is arguably a deterministic way of viewing happiness, there are links between certain hormones and subjective experience. For example, having lower levels of the hormonal mood regulator serotonin may lead to depression. The next section of this chapter explores how happiness is measured. But before moving on to that, please take some time out for Pause for Reflection 6.2.

Pause for Reflection 6.2

Happiness is a complex concept. Take some time to think about how you would measure it. How might you find out if someone is happy (or not)? Would you use subjective measures (such as asking them how they feel) or objective measures (such as observing their facial expressions for signs of happiness)? Or perhaps a combination of both?

Measuring happiness

Due to the increased interest in happiness in recent decades, there are now many ways in which it may be measured. A lot of research has been focused on measuring happiness, exploring why some people (and nations) are happier than others (BBC News, 2015). Questions about happiness appear in many surveys which aim to find out about quality of life or well-being. For example, the UK Office for National Statistics' (ONS) Household Survey includes the following question: 'Overall, how happy did you feel yesterday?' (World Economic Forum, 2015).

Happiness can be explored subjectively by, for example, asking people how they feel (emotional states and affect), or objectively by, for example, asking people to evaluate their levels of satisfaction with life. Most people, when asked, are able to make an assessment of their own state of happiness using either subjective or objective means (Daniel-González et al., 2023). Happiness as a subjective construct, and levels of happiness, can be determined by asking people how happy they are on, for example, a scale of 1 to 10, or asking about what makes them happy (Veehoven, 2003). Of course, the answers will vary considerably depending on who you ask, where and when. Forgeard et al. (2011) point out the appeal of using questions about how happy people are – it is a simple means of measurement. Surveys might ask single-item questions such as 'are you happy?', 'when was the last time you felt happy?' or 'how happy are you today?' A widely used single-item question about subjective levels of happiness was employed in Gyasi et al.'s (2023) Ghanaian study: 'Over the past four weeks, have you been a happy person?', with four possible responses – all of the time, most of the time, little of the time and none of the time. One of the questions in the Indonesian Family Life Survey is specifically about happiness: 'Taken all together, how would you say you are these days: very happy, pretty happy, not too happy, or very unhappy?' (Sujarwoto, 2021: 680). Similar single-unit measurements are used in surveys in many different countries.

More complex measurements include several related questions (multi-item questionnaires) (Steptoe, 2019). Happiness research conducted in Japan conceptualized happiness in an objective way by asking people to evaluate their happiness on a 10-point scale, where 0 equated to least happy, and 10 equated to most happy (Tsuruta et al., 2019). However, it is not possible to ascertain the basis on which people decide to respond to such questions, or the reasons why they might answer as they do, so it is not an exact science. Any such questions are open to interpretation by the participants, and individual, subjective assessments will likely result in any number of interpretations of happiness. Consequently, some researchers have developed more objective, quantifiable means of measurement (Forgeard et al., 2011).

Like well-being, happiness can be measured using subjective (self-reporting) or objective (observing physiological states) means (Green et al., 2019). However, the research is dominated by subjective measures of happiness where people self-evaluate and self-report typically by using survey scales. Another challenge with measurement is the oft-used strategy of asking people to retrospectively assess their levels of happiness – for example, 'how happy were you last week?' This relies on people's memory and may not, therefore, be a good measure of how happy they actually were at the time.

Krys et al. (2021) point out that societal happiness is often measured by asking individuals how satisfied they are with their lives and then extrapolating that to an indicator of the happiness of everyone. Like others, Krys et al. demonstrate how levels of personal happiness correlate with levels of individualism, which is typically a result of how happiness is measured (using individual constructs). In their paper they talk about different types of happiness, including *family* inter-dependent happiness: 'the collective happiness of one's family and the extent to which one's family is in harmony with other families and groups in one's community' (Krys et al., 2021: 2199). In their study involving over 13,000 participants from fifty countries they also measured collective types of happiness such as family interdependent happiness and family life satisfaction, and found that these were predicted more by cultural factors than by individualism. See Box 6.3 for more detail about individualism and societal happiness.

Box 6.3: Individualism and societal happiness (Krys et al., cited in Krys et al., 2021: 2198)

'Individualism promotes societal happiness if it adopts the form of *the open society*. Four attitude orientations constituting open society: (1) tolerance, (2) trust, (3) civic engagement, and (4) non-materialism tend to benefit society as a whole, but do not directly and substantially promote individual satisfaction. Individuals endorsing open society attitudes are not considerably more satisfied than prejudiced, suspicious, uninvolved, and materialistic members of the same society, but societies in which open society attitudes are prevalent report greater happiness than closed societies.'

Happiness scales can be cross-culturally validated, as in the case of Gyasi et al. (2023), who used a five-point scale for Ghanaian older adults to self-rate their personal levels of happiness. However, critiques of subjective measures of happiness centre on their individualistic nature and the fact that they promote a politics of personal behaviour. Many measures of happiness are rooted in Eurocentric and American notions of what happiness is, which tend to privilege individualistic aspects such as personal achievements and life satisfaction and pay little heed to the values espoused by more collective societies (Krys et al., 2021). Similarly, White (2017: 121) argues that the attention given to happiness reflects 'the erosion of the social in late capitalist modernity'; criticizing its individualistic nature, she points to collectivist societies that pay more attention to societal well-being than individual well-being, and highlights the importance of social inclusion and cohesion for individual happiness. Krys et al. (2021) also note how certain regions of the world, such as Africa, Eastern Europe, Latin America, the Middle East and South Asia, are under-represented in the happiness research. A similar point is made by Beida et al. (2017), who are critical of the attention to happiness being a 'northern' or 'western' preoccupation and note the profusion of research from Europe and the global north at the exclusion of the global majority. This may be because happiness is less of a priority in situations where food, shelter and safety take precedence. There are some exceptions, however. For example, Bhattacharyya et al. (2019) have explored how India might improve population happiness. Drawing on evidence from happier Nordic countries, Bhattacharyya et al. (2019: 28) make the following recommendations for achieving a 'Happy India':

- Working towards a more equitable society
- Developing a trustworthy social support system where each citizen has a moral responsibility
- Instilling a spirit of generosity and voluntary social service through formation of community self-service groups in both rural and urban societies
- Making environmental concerns a priority
- Transparency and institutional integrity which restores faith of the public in government
- Enhancement of public spending on health and medical infrastructure

Burns and Crisp (2022) note that the research on happiness, although burgeoning, has some significant limitations, including the lack of an agreed definition of happiness and the lack of clear/consistent indicators or measures. Most importantly, they point to the fact that many studies emphasize (and assume) that happiness is an outcome equally valued by everyone, when that is not necessarily the case. Other challenges with measuring happiness include its association with other phenomena, which can lead to confounding and reverse causation (Steptoe, 2019). Psychologist Martin Seligman (2011) considers happiness a problematic construct for meaningful research since, he argues, it does not capture the 'true multifaceted nature of human flourishing' (Forgeard et al., 2011: 96). Notwithstanding the complications involved in researching and measuring happiness, many would argue that it is important we continue to try to do so. In fact, Wang et al. (2022: 2) argue that 'efforts to assess and improve happiness might help countries to understand and improve what really matters to people'. Box 6.4 details two examples of measures of happiness: the Subjective Happiness Scale and the Oxford Happiness Questionnaire.

Earlier in this chapter we noted the paradigm shift that has occurred in this area (a shift also reflected in Chapter 5 when we discussed the increased focus on non-monetary measures of success). Happiness indices now offer a way of measuring quality of life outside of economic means. Bhutan led the way in establishing a non-monetary system of measuring success, and it now has a Gross National Happiness Index (as distinct from the more common gross national product measure [GNP]). Other countries have followed suit. Happiness is also measured globally, whereby countries are compared to one another. According to the World Happiness Report for 2023, Finland was the happiest country in the world (as it had been for the previous six years) (Helliwell et al., 2023). The Report has been published every year since 2012. It evaluates happiness using measures in relation to six different areas: social support, gross domestic product per capita, healthy life expectancy, freedom to make your own choices, generosity of the general population, and absence of corruption (World Population Review, 2023). The least happy countries in 2023 were Afghanistan and Lebanon. Notably, the measurements used in the World Happiness Report differ from typical subjective measures of individual happiness such as those detailed in Box 6.4. In contrast to subjective experiences of happiness, the Report assesses what might be considered 'determinants' of happiness in society – things that need to be in place for happiness to be realized. The 'open society' concept discussed in Box 6.3 is reflected in some of the Report's areas of measurement, for example in relation to social support and absence of corruption.*

---

* For more detail, see https://worldhappiness.report.

Box 6.4: Measures of happiness – two examples

Subjective Happiness Scale (Lyubomirsky and Lepper, 1999)
For each of the following statements and/or questions, please circle the point on the scale that you feel is most appropriate in describing you:

1. In general, I consider myself:
   not a very happy person 1 2 3 4 5 6 7 a very happy person
2. Compared with most of my peers, I consider myself:
   less happy 1 2 3 4 5 6 7 more happy
3. Some people are generally very happy. They enjoy life regardless of what is going on, getting the most out of everything. To what extent does this characterization describe you?
   not at all 1 2 3 4 5 6 7 a great deal
4. Some people are generally not very happy. Although they are not depressed, they never seem as happy as they might be. To what extent does this characterization describe you?
   not at all 1 2 3 4 5 6 7 a great deal

Oxford Happiness Questionnaire – Short Scale (Hills and Argyle, 2002).
The OHQ is completed by scoring each statement according to how much a person agrees or disagrees with it, using a code from 1 = strongly disagree, to 6 = strongly agree. The following statements comprise the shorter version of the questionnaire (the full version has twenty-nine items).

1. I don't feel particularly pleased with the way I am
2. I feel that life is very rewarding
3. I am well satisfied about everything in my life
4. I don't think I look attractive
5. I find beauty in some things
6. I can fit in everything I want to
7. I feel fully mentally alert
8. I do not have particularly happy memories of the past

For the longer version of this and details about how to complete both versions, see the Oxford Happiness Questionnaire (Hills and Argyle, 2002).

Case Study 6: Social media, happiness and health

Social media influences our ideas about what it means to be happy and how we might attain happiness. It also influences our feelings of happiness, impacting positively and negatively on our subjective experience and mood states. It can enhance or reduce our happiness and well-being depending on how we use it (Kross et al., 2021). Engaging with social media might boost our happiness by raising our self-esteem through positive feedback or improving our mood if we see or engage with content that is life-affirming, encouraging or simply funny. But the downside of social media is that it tends to be dominated by discourse about perfect lives, promoting cultural expectations and normative standards around attaining happiness and what it means to be happy (Dolan, 2019). This, in turn, is linked to consumption. Social media also encourages consumption in the pursuit of happiness.

For young people, problematic social media use has been associated with lower levels of happiness, which are in turn associated with difficulties sleeping and lower levels of physical activity (Bozzola et al., 2022; Zhang et al., 2022a). Social media is pervasive, constantly available and its content is easily tailored to the individual's interests through hidden algorithms which encourage engagement and use. Problematic social media use refers to the growing issue of addiction to social media, which is especially prevalent in adolescents, although a distinction is made between disordered social media use (by those who seem to be addicted to it) and 'high-engaging non-disordered' use (Van den Eijnden et al., 2016: 478). Evidence suggests that disordered social media use has a negative impact on physical, mental and social health. This is exacerbated by the portrayal of 'perfect' lives. Conversely, non-disordered social media use can have many positive effects, including boosting social interaction, making friends, providing support and sharing common interests, which, in turn, have a positive impact on happiness (Chen, 2017). Whilst social media can be a social lifeline for some people, it might also bring problems such as cyberbullying, which can lead to significant psychological harm. A meta-analysis carried out by Cunningham et al. (2021) found that, among young people, the likelihood of experiencing symptoms of depression was higher with problematic social media use.

Summary

Krys et al. (2021: 2210) argue that 'ultimately there are many ways of conceptualizing and living a happy [healthy] and good life'. As pointed out in Chapter 1, Saracci (1997) criticized the WHO's definition of health as having more to do with happiness than with health. He argued that health and happiness are distinct and 'have no fixed relationship with each other', going on to state that although health is arguably a right, 'no one can guarantee the right of happiness' (Saracci, 1997: 1049). Nevertheless, as we have seen in this chapter, happiness continues to be of interest on the assumption that micro- and macro-level policy can be developed that will increase the potential for happiness to be experienced and expressed. Wang et al. (2022: 13) point out that 'both happiness and health are important indicators for a prosperous society'. Yet, as Steptoe (2019: 352) observes, 'many questions remain unresolved in this fast-moving field'. Finally, an editorial in *The Lancet* (2016) argued that we need to find out more about the association between health and happiness in order to understand how we can promote sustainable development. It also insisted that 'indices of overall well-being must not obscure the need for ongoing progress in reducing disease, mental illness and premature death. Without life, there is no happiness to be realised' (The Lancet, 2016: 1251).

Further reading

For further detail about happiness and health see Steptoe, A. (2019) Happiness and health. *Annual Review of Public Health*, 40, 339–59, https://doi.org/10.1146/annurev-publhealth-040218-044150

Author's summary: 'Research into the relationship between happiness and health is developing rapidly, exploring the possibility that impaired happiness is not only a consequence of ill health but also a potential contributor to disease risk. Happiness encompasses several constructs, including affective well-being (feelings of joy and pleasure), eudemonic well-being (sense of meaning and purpose in life), and evaluative well-being (life satisfaction). Happiness is generally associated with reduced mortality in prospective observational studies, albeit with several discrepant results. Confounding and reverse causation are major concerns. Associations with morbidity and disease prognosis have also been identified for a limited range of health conditions. The mechanisms potentially linking happiness with health include lifestyle factors, such as physical activity and dietary choice, and biological processes, involving neuroendocrine, inflammatory, and metabolic pathways. Interventions have yet to demonstrate substantial, sustained improvements in subjective well-being or direct impact on physical health outcomes. Nevertheless, this field shows great potential, with the promise of establishing a favourable effect on population health.'

7
Creating Health

Chapter aims

- To critically consider the question 'what makes people healthy?'
- To introduce and discuss the theory of salutogenesis
- To describe and explore asset-based approaches to health

Introduction

In this chapter we are concerned with the question 'what makes people healthy?' So far, this book has considered several different ideas about perspectives about what health is and what determines it. In this chapter we turn our attention to what *creates* health. As well as giving due attention to action on the social determinants of health as discussed in Chapter 3, this chapter focuses more heavily on salutogenic perspectives and asset-based approaches to creating health. We start by briefly discussing policy approaches to tackling the social determinants of health, then move on to Aaron Antonovsky's theory of salutogenesis. The discussion will draw upon global research and evidence from the wider literature about the effectiveness of salutogenic approaches to health, and suggest how these might be maximized for health gain, before moving on to consider asset-based approaches. Before you read any further please take some time out to do Pause for Reflection 7.1.

> **Pause for Reflection 7.1**
>
> This chapter considers how health is created. Creating health requires us to think about what health *is*, so you might want to reflect on some of the discussion in the preceding chapters to frame your ideas. What do you think is the way to health? What factors do you think are essential for health to exist and be maintained? How might health be created or achieved?

Creating health

The first thing we will consider in answer to the question 'what makes people healthy?' is how we might tackle the social determinants of health. Marmot et al. (2020: 149) point out how the health of billions of people is 'made worse by social conditions they had no part in creating'. So, logic tells us that tackling these social conditions will be a means of creating better health. As outlined in Chapter 4, health is determined by many different things and, to a large extent, is socially determined through the social structures and environments in which we live our everyday lives.

Of course, tackling such determinants requires, above all things, political will. Better health has long been the focus of public policy. Many people argue that social justice (or fairness) should be the foundation for developing policy that aims to improve health. A large body of work led by Sir Michael Marmot under the Commission on the Social Determinants of Health has resulted in many publications, including a review of health inequalities in England. As a result of that work Marmot et al. (2020: 151) made the six policy recommendations listed in Chapter 4 (see page 89 above). Many people, including Marmot et al. (2020), strongly advocate for proportionate universalism as a means of tackling health inequity and creating better health for those who suffer most. Proportionate universalism is about directing attention and resources to those who are most in need, with the aim of improving the health of the worst off but also reducing health inequalities across the social gradient. Focusing efforts on those most in need is a means of creating better health, as is tackling health inequities more generally (Zhang et al., 2022c). Examples of proportionate universalism include progressive taxation and redistribution of resources.

The focus on healthy public policy has been a key theme in the World Health Organization's health promotion agenda, which has championed the 'health in all policies' approach in recognition that health is a cross-policy concern, not just confined to healthcare. Healthy public policy is concerned with 'positive outcomes and solutions to problems' (Lindström and Eriksson, 2009: 21). In order to create health, therefore, policy must focus on meeting unmet needs, tackling low income and its consequences such as food and energy poverty, and addressing lack of access to healthcare and education (Kiran and Pinto, 2016). With regard to creating health in the European context, 'a wide range of policies can help to influence this, ranging from employment and social protection strategies to the food we eat and how much we walk rather than drive' (Wismar et al., 2018: xvii).

The theory of salutogenesis

The term salutogenesis comes from two Latin words: salus meaning *health* and genesis meaning *emergence* (Röhrich et al., 2021). Harrop et al. (2007: 46) point out that the term also means 'giving birth to health', since 'the word salutogenesis is itself derived from a combination of "salus" meaning health and "genesis" meaning "giving birth"'. Sociologist Aaron Antonovsky (1996) introduced the theory of salutogenesis in the late 1970s and refined it some ten years later. The theory resulted from research that Antonovsky carried out on Israeli women who had survived incarceration in concentration camps in the Second World War. He found that 29 per cent of the women survivors in his research had 'managed to survive the horrors of the camps without any apparent psychological insult' (Röhrich et al., 2021: 594). Antonovksy wanted to know how these women stayed relatively healthy despite extreme adversity. He identified three key factors: 'the ability for people to understand what happens around them; to what extent they were able to manage the situation on their own or through significant others in their social network; and the ability to find meaning in the situation' (Eriksson and Lindström, 2005: 460). He therefore suggested that we should be looking at what creates health, i.e. why some people are able to stay healthy whilst other people are not, and particularly why this might be the case when people are faced with similar sets of adverse circumstances. Salutogenesis, then, is fundamentally concerned with 'what factors support health' (Svalastog et al., 2017: 432), or how health might be generated or created rather than how ill health might be prevented (Skovdal, 2013). With its focus on the conditions that create health, salutogenesis challenges the pathogenic nature of the medical model of health discussed in Chapter 1 (Woodall and Cross, 2022). As such, Skovdal (2013: 159) defines salutogenesis as 'an approach focusing on factors that support human health and well-being, rather than on factors that cause disease'. Box 7.1 lists the assumptions underpinning pathogenic approaches to health that exist in opposition to the principles of salutogenesis.

Box 7.1: Assumptions underpinning pathogenic approaches to health (after Antonovsky, 1984, cited in Green et al., 2019: 92)

- the tendency to think dichotomously about people, classifying them as either healthy or diseased
- a focus on disease states or risk factors
- the search for a cause or multifactorial causes
- the assumption that stressors are bad
- mounting wars against specific diseases
- ignoring the factors associated with wellness

The basic principle underpinning salutogenesis is that health is always in a state of flux. This is characterized by Antonovsky (1984: 117) as the '"health-ease-dis-ease" continuum'. The idea is that people continually move back and forth along this continuum throughout their lifespan, either towards health or towards disease, never really settling at one end of the continuum or the other. The theory suggests that no one is ever 100 per cent healthy, rather health and illness co-exist (Röhrich et al., 2021). Antonovsky (1996) maintained that it was impossible for us to achieve full health given that we are all biological beings with physical bodies vulnerable to disease and deterioration (Cross et al., 2021a). Thus, 'salutogenesis recognizes aspects of health within a person regardless of the state and extent of the disease' (Röhrich et al., 2021: 594) (see Box 7.2).

Box 7.2: Key points in the development of salutogenesis (after Eriksson and Lindström, 2008: 192–3)

1940s–1960s: A group of Israeli women survived the Holocaust. Three decades later this group would become the subjects of the first study of salutogenesis.

1970s: A paradigm shift from the pathogenic to the salutogenic perspective on health. Antonovsky introduces the concept of 'sense of coherence'.

1980s: Antonovsky revises and develops salutogenic theory. Salutogenic research is still limited, with few publications.

1990s: Increasing interest in salutogenesis and a corresponding increase in research and publications. First international research courses on salutogenesis in Scandinavia.

2000s: The salutogenic approach takes hold and research expands further. By 2007 the sense of coherence concept is used in forty-four languages.

2010 to date: Further increased interest in, and research on, salutogenesis. The first edition of the international *Handbook of Salutogenesis* is published in 2016, followed by the second edition in 2022.

Sense of coherence

Antonovsky suggested that the women who survived their concentration camp experience apparently psychologically intact displayed what he referred to as 'hardiness' (Röhrich et al., 2021). It was this that led to the development of the sense of coherence concept. According to Antonovsky, how we see the world (our perspective) influences our capacity to cope with and manage life's stressors (Eriksson and Lindström, 2008). This, in turn, impacts on our health through two mechanisms: our sense of coherence and our 'general resistance resources'. We will return to the concept of general resistance resources in a moment, but first let us consider sense of coherence in more detail.

Sense of coherence is one of the key constructs in salutogenesis and is about 'understanding, managing and making sense of change' (Wills, 2023: 6). It can also be understood as 'a secondary appraisal [of a stressful situation] that facilitates the exploration of resources available to the individual to deal with [that] stressful situation' (Braun-Lewensohn and Mayer, 2020: 668). The three key components of sense of coherence, as theorized by Antonovksy, are comprehensibility (the cognitive element – how we understand our world and make sense of it), meaningfulness (the motivational element – how we feel about this) and manageability (the instrumental/behavioural element – how we cope with the challenges of life) (Eriksson and Lindström, 2005; Sidell, 2010). As Green et al. (2019: 92) argue, 'salutogenesis focuses on the factors associated with successful coping, which are envisaged as buffers mitigating the effects of stressors'.

Antonovsky argued that people with a stronger sense of coherence are more likely to be able to achieve better health (Cross and Woodall, 2024). Sense of coherence is about how we respond to different stressors, which can include, for example, 'microbial, physical, chemical, psychosocial stressors' (Green et al., 2019: 92). Having a sense of coherence contributes to a person's resilience when facing adversity or stressors (Röhrich et al., 2021). As observed by Eriksson and Lindström (2008: 196), 'a strong Sense of Coherence helps us to identify and use the resources needed to solve emerging problems'. Sense of coherence increases with age, although it is not clear whether this is because healthy people live longer or because people with a stronger sense of coherence stay healthier for longer (Eriksson and Lindström, 2005). In short, 'the Sense of Coherence construct reflects a person's capacity to respond [and adapt] to stressful situations' (Eriksson and Lindström, 2005: 460) whatever those situations might be.

Generalized resistance resources

The other key concept in salutogenesis is 'generalized resistance resources', which refers to a range of factors that provide some kind of support for living life in a coherent way (Lindström and Eriksson, 2006). Generalized resistance resources can be conceptualized as internal or external to a person, and can be material or non-material (Harrop et al., 2007). Such factors include psychosocial, biological and material forms of support, for example resilience, relationships with others, healthy behaviours, good genetics, money and employment. Other factors include commitment, cultural stability and religion/philosophy (Eriksson and Lindström, 2005). In addition, a person's ability to identify and use the resources that are available to them is determined by their sense of coherence (Braun-Lewensohn and Mayer, 2020). Generalized resistance resources provide support for a sense of coherence, hence people with a greater sense of coherence and access to a variety of generalized resistance resources will do better than people with less of both.

Research on salutogenesis

There has been a burgeoning of research into salutogenesis over the past few decades, most of which has been done in the global north. In this section we consider some examples from across the world. A systematic review of eating behaviours/habits and sense of coherence has shown that the two are positively linked (Veiga et al., 2022).

A weak sense of coherence was related to 'an increase in fast eating, an irregular diet and an excess of food at night supper', whilst a stronger sense of coherence was associated with healthier eating patterns (Veiga et al., 2022: 2519). Other studies have shown similar findings with regards to sense of coherence and other types of healthy behaviour, such as a greater likelihood of being physically active, better oral health practices and the increased likelihood of not smoking. International research carried out during the COVID-19 pandemic in nine countries (Israel, Italy, Spain, the Netherlands, Germany, Switzerland, Austria, Brazil and the United States) found that a sense of coherence was a key coping resource and concluded that a strong sense of coherence is necessary 'for health and survival during times of global and local crises' (Mana et al., 2021: 2). A special issue on salutogenesis and coping published in 2020 in the *International Journal of Research in Public Health* included several papers reporting on research involving different age groups and ethnic groups in different countries. Some of this work is summarized here:

- Moksnes and Espnes (2020) carried out research with Norwegian adolescents examining sense of coherence (SOC) and relationship stress and concluded that sense of coherence is a major coping resource in the context of depression and mental well-being. 'The findings provide support for the significant role of SOC as a coping resource, especially in relation to adolescents' mental health' (2020: 1).
- Braun-Lewensohn et al. (2020) explored the coping resources and mental health of Syrian women living in a refugee camp in Greece and showed that sense of coherence is vital for good adaptation. Sense of coherence was found to mediate appraisal of dangers and the amount of time spent in the camp.
- In a study by Barnard and Furtak (2020) of volunteers in South Africa, sense of coherence in the form of an inner drive and a calling was shown to be integral to psychological resilience and well-being. The research found that a characteristic work–life orientation was at the root of

the volunteers' resilience, which enabled them to cope with and adjust to the challenges of volunteering in that context.

- Research from the Democratic Republic of Congo on coping, sense of coherence, burnout and work engagement found a positive relationship between coping and sense of coherence, and that the latter was negatively associated with work engagement and burnout (Mitonga-Monga and Mayer, 2020). The authors suggest that an employee who has a high level of coping, a high sense of coherence and a low level of burnout is more likely to be an engaged, productive and performing employee.

As illustrated here, there is a lot of empirical support for salutogenesis. It appears to be relevant to human experience cross-culturally, although it is acknowledged that there is a relative dearth of salutogenic research in the global south compared to the global north (Mitonga-Monga and Mayer, 2020). See Box 7.3 for further details.

Box 7.3: Salutogenesis – a universal concept?

Antonovsky contended that the concept of salutogenesis is universal, applicable cross-culturally and not dependent on any particular worldview. He argued that 'seeing the world as comprehensible, manageable, and meaningful would facilitate the selection of culturally appropriate and situationally efficacious resources and behaviours' (Antonovsky, 1996: 174). Wallerstein similarly pointed out that sense of coherence eliminates the cultural bias of the concept of 'control', which has typically promoted individual decision making at the expense of the group (Wallerstein, cited in Harrop et al., 2007: 48). A systemic review by Eriksson and Lindström (2005) also concurs that sense of coherence is cross-culturally applicable for ascertaining how people cope with life and stay healthy.

Salutogenic approaches to health

In contrast to salutogenic approaches, pathogenic approaches to health focus on what causes ill health and disease. Such approaches are of course important in terms of prevention, treatment and cure, and they have a significant role to play in the promotion of maximum health experience. Salutogenic theory does not refute this (Taylor et al., 2014). However, as discussed, Antonovsky (1996) proposed that we should take a broader perspective in order to find out what makes people healthy. Salutogenic approaches thus emphasize factors that 'create and support health, well-being, happiness and meaning in life' (Gregg and O'Hara, 2007: 14). See Box 7.4 for a definition of a salutogenic approach.

Box 7.4: A salutogenic approach (Taylor et al., 2014: 285)

'A salutogenic approach includes focusing on perceived health and happiness [see Chapter 6], purpose in life, spiritual connections, social support, a healthy ecosystem, physical resilience, optimism and hope, and the ability to experience emotions, in addition to addressing risk factors for poor health such as poverty, unemployment, disparity, powerlessness, isolation and discrimination.'

In a review of resilience, coping and salutogenic approaches to maintaining and generating health, Harrop et al. (2007) found that there were two main types of salutogenic intervention discussed in the wider literature. Firstly, 'approaches aimed at strengthening resources (e.g. self-management skills, community networks)', and, secondly, 'approaches aimed at creating meaning and order (e.g. interventions to increase perceptions of control, and therapy interventions)' (Harrop et al., 2007: 10). Braun-Lewensohn and Mayer (2020: 667) also discuss coping in relation to life's stressors, arguing that 'the characteristics of an individual and the way [they] appraise a situation are important elements for [their] well-being in the aftermath of a stressful or conflictual encounter'. Salutogenic approaches emphasize people's ability to adapt and access/use available resources to create health (Bhattacharya et al., 2020). The 'salutogenic orientation' includes the need to nurture capacities to increase health as well as the requirement to foster resources for health (Bauer et al., 2020); it is also concerned with identifying protective factors for health (Cassetti et al., 2019). As argued by Röhrich et al. (2021), this kind of perspective is really important in the context of chronic diseases, which are on the increase globally. Preventive measures and means of promoting and maximizing health are vital for those living with chronic disease. Röhrich et al. (2021) contend that, alongside medicine, alternative creative approaches are required to improve treatment and resiliency. As they point out, we will all get sick at some point, and 'a person's vulnerability to chronic disease can increase over the course of an extended lifetime as a consequence of lifestyle choices and activities, socioeconomic situation, environmental influences'; furthermore, 'the onset and development of chronic disease often increases vulnerability to, and the likelihood of, contracting other conditions' (Röhrich et al., 2021: 593). Of course, some people are able to maintain positivity and well-being in spite of living with chronic illness (Meldgaard et al., 2022). Danish research on people living with Type 2 diabetes (Meldgaard et al., 2022) presented three key findings: First, despite living with a chronic illness, having the condition was viewed as manageable due to general optimism. Second, social support was hugely beneficial as a way of sharing the burden. Third, having an open dialogue and being able to talk about the difficulties of having Type 2 diabetes was also important. The authors argued that these three findings 'may reinforce each other in an upward spiral and enhance the sense of coherence' (Meldgaard et al., 2022: 1).

Despite the appeal of salutogenesis, and the evidence for the value of having a high sense of coherence and access to generalized resistance resources, there is still more work to be done to strengthen the knowledge and evidence base. Bauer et al. (2020: 187) suggest that this work should address four key conceptual issues:

1. The overall salutogenic model of health
2. The sense of coherence (SOC) concept
3. The design of salutogenic interventions and change processes in complex systems
4. The applications of salutogenesis beyond the health sector

Box 7.5 expands on each of these in more detail.

Box 7.5: The future of salutogenesis – four key issues (Bauer et al., 2020: 193)

1. 'The original salutogenic model of health needs to be advanced by adding an additional positive health continuum and a direct path of positive health development operating independently of stressors. This expansion of the theory and of the model will support health promotion researchers and practitioners in efforts to address the full spectrum of the human health experience.
2. For a better understanding of the SOC, we encourage alternative approaches to the conceptualization and measurement of the SOC, including qualitative research. A high priority is to develop better understanding of the origins of SOC in the earliest life years. In addition, the idea to re-examine the original data analysed by Antonovsky is being explored. Would we, in the modern context, interpret his interviews in a similar way, or would additional insight into the SOC emerge?
3. To purposefully design salutogenic interventions and change processes, we suggest the development of explicit salutogenic intervention theories that build on and integrate key elements of salutogenesis, including strengthening resources, promoting coherent (i.e. comprehensible, manageable, meaningful) life experiences and positive health outcomes.
4. It would be fruitful to apply salutogenesis beyond traditional, individual health issues, as other fields can profit from this concept and as we can learn from such

fields for health research. The case of SOC in inter-group relations demonstrates that we need to more fully examine the differential benefits and potential harm of SOC on the individual, group and intergroup as well as organizational and system levels.'

Salutogenic approaches to health sit well with asset-based approaches: both are concerned with what builds, sustains and restores health, and the factors that 'fortify individuals' and communities' health determinants and resources' (Röhrich et al., 2021: 591). The next section considers asset-based approaches to health. Before reading any further, please take some time out to complete Pause for Reflection 7.2.

Pause for Reflection 7.2

What do you know about asset-based approaches to health? Using the internet, take some time to find out what they are and see if you can summarize what you find. What are the key features of asset-based approaches and why are they pertinent to health? Try to identify some examples of these approaches and determine how they create or enable health.

Asset-based approaches to health

Asset-based approaches to health exist in opposition to deficit-based approaches. Deficit-based approaches tend to focus on risk factors and what people are doing wrong, what is not working or is missing. In contrast, asset-based approaches 'look at the resources of individuals and communities and how these can be harnessed to improve health and well-being' (Skovdal, 2013: 89), and 'seek to positively mobilise the strengths, capabilities, and resources of individuals and communities' (Astbury et al., 2021: 1257).

Asset-based approaches focus more on what makes people healthy rather than what makes them unwell. The Glasgow Centre for Population Health (2011: 2) defines assets as 'the collective resources which individuals and communities have at their disposal, which protect against negative health outcomes and promote health status'. *Health* assets refer to anything that enables people to attain better health and well-being (Ziglio et al., 2017). Asset-based models fit nicely with salutogenesis because they emphasize the potential of people to promote their own health (Kawachi, 2010); they have thus become 'increasingly popular as a way to tackle health inequalities by empowering people in more disadvantaged communities to use local resources and increase control over health and its determinants' (Cassetti et al., 2019: 15).

Assets may exist at many levels: the individual level, the community level or the societal/system level. Earlier in this chapter we talked about hardiness in reference to Antonovsky's work. In the literature, hardiness is often conceptualized as *resilience*, which is widely viewed as an important asset (or resource) for health, protecting against adversity. However, there are those who caution against paying too much attention to resilience at the individual level, given the potential of this to distract from the social determinants of health and the tendency to blame individuals for not being resilient enough when they do not thrive. For example, Friedli (2013) argues that such approaches focus on individual psychosocial factors at the expense of the economic, material and structural issues that impact on health (see the discussion in Chapter 4). Resilience, however, is not just evident at the individual level. Health sociologist Ziglio and colleagues (2017) argue that it can be cultivated at community and system levels as well. They provide a framework that considers four different types of resilience capacity. See Box 7.6 for more details.

Ziglio et al. argue that the three different levels (individual, community and system) and the four types of resilience capacity seen in Box 7.6 should form the basis for designing healthy public policy.

In addition to resilience there are many other assets that can be drawn upon to create, maintain and maximize health. Morgan and Ziglio (2007: 17) state that a health asset can

---

Box 7.6: Types of resilience (Ziglio et al., 2017: 789)

'*Adaptive* capacity refers to the ability of individuals, communities and systems to adjust to disturbances and shocks.

Absorptive capacity is the ability to absorb and effectively manage and recover from adverse conditions, drawing on available skills, assets and resources.

Anticipatory capacity is the ability to predict and reduce disturbances and risks by means of proactive action to minimize vulnerability.

Transformative capacity applies mainly to systems: it refers to their ability to transform their structures and means of operating to better address change and uncertainty. It is the ability to develop (new) systems that are more suited to new conditions.'

---

be 'any factor (or resource) which enhances the ability of individuals, groups, communities, populations, social systems and/or institutions to maintain and sustain health and well-being and to help reduce health inequities'. Community assets include things like mutual trust and solidarity as well as good social networks, all of which have been shown to be beneficial for health and well-being (Ziglio et al., 2017). Irby et al. (2021) point out the value of cultural assets and argue that it is vital to work with communities to design culturally appropriate interventions to improve health and tackle inequalities. They refer specifically to American Indian communities in North Carolina, who experience inequalities in terms of poverty, education, chronic disease, access to healthcare and overall quality of life. Box 7.7 details some further health assets.

Ideas about control are also significant. As Ziglio et al. (2017: 789) argue, 'the level of control (or lack of it) that a person has over his or her life has been shown to be a key factor in the social determination of health and health inequities'. So, having a feeling of control is also an important asset for health.

Box 7.7: Health assets (Skovdal, 2013: 89)

'Health assets can include factors from across the range of the determinants of health, including genetic make-up, economic and social conditions, environmental conditions, health behaviour, and use of health and other services', as well as 'family and friendship networks, intergenerational solidarity, community cohesion, environmental resources necessary for promoting physical, mental and social health, employment security and opportunities for voluntary service, affinity groups (such as mutual aid), religious tolerance and harmony, life-long learning, safe and pleasant housing, political democracy and participation opportunities, social justice and enhancing equity.'

Having established that asset-based approaches are important for the creation of health it is necessary to consider how they might be operationalized. A systematic scoping review by Cassetti et al. (2019) examined 30 papers that used an asset-based approach and identified three key approaches to mobilizing assets: connecting assets, raising awareness of assets and enabling assets to thrive. Each of these approaches was effective in making a difference. Asset-based approaches can therefore be viewed as critical alternatives to approaches that focus on what is lacking or deficient. They aim to promote health and well-being as well as tackling health inequalities by utilizing the resources, skills and strengths that already exist within communities, as identified by the communities themselves (Astbury et al., 2021). As Green et al. (2019: 125) argue, 'to adopt an assets-based approach is to recognize the experience, skills, strengths, knowledge and potential that already exist in a group or community and how these (may) contribute to the support of health and well-being'.

Earlier in this chapter we considered the role of public policy in creating health. In a published case study, Lindström and Eriksson (2009) applied a salutogenic framework to public policy in an unnamed European country experiencing system change, ethnic conflict and financial crisis. They argued that these problems had put the national sense of coherence in the country under threat. Addressing the question of how 'health public policy [can] be made comprehensible, manageable and meaningful to all involved' (Lindström and Eriksson, 2009: 20), they highlighted the importance of identifying what is meaningful to the population concerned by engaging with that population rather than imposing ideas upon it about what is important.

Pérez-Wilson et al. (2021) suggest that salutogenesis and the health assets model should be integrated in order to fully develop their potential for health improvement and to create a more coherent approach. They argue that salutogenic theory needs to be 'more action-oriented' and that the assets model needs to be 'more theoretical' (2021: 884). Whilst Pérez-Wilson et al. do propose a synergistic model that brings the two together (see the paper for further details), clearly more work is needed to take this field forward, in keeping with the four key recommendations presented earlier from Bauer et al. (2020).

Case Study 7: Asset-mapping in rural Ecuador (adapted from Bates et al., 2019)

Maps are often used with and in communities as a basis for establishing assets in existence in the location in which the community lives. In this case study, the authors worked with members of four different rural communities in Ecuador to provide an alternative cartography to the existing maps that 'privileg[e] the interests of the global North and ... authorize (neo)colonial approaches' (p. 228). Bates et al. argue that, historically, maps have been used in the global south to identify deficits and problems which require intervention from the global north, thereby reflecting a certain worldview that is not necessarily representative of the people who live in the area or region. The argument for drawing up alternative maps is rooted in the creation of new and different discourses of politics and power (Barney, 2009).

The authors worked with people from four communities: Bellamaria and Chaquizhca in Loja province, a mountainous region; and Roi Mariano and Pechichal in Manabi province, a coastal region. The maps were produced as part of an asset-mapping process derived from the Asset-Based Community Development (ABCD) approach, which 'relies on a community identifying its assets that enable health and development, rather than the needs-oriented approach' (p. 233), focusing on the abilities of communities to find their own solutions to their problems instead of having solutions forced upon them. 'The underlying philosophy driving the ABCD strategy is the belief that each individual has capacities, abilities, and gifts, and that communities are strongest when each individual has opportunities to share these with others' (p. 233).

The process began with appreciative interviews and focus groups within each community. Participants were asked to make maps of the assets and resources they valued, prompted by the question 'Draw a map that includes what you think is important or significant about your community' (p. 234). The community members identified several assets, including shared resources such as buildings and roads, and natural resources such as forest, river and coast, as well as foul, fish and livestock. They also identified human resources – prominent community figures, and the talents and skills of specific community members. The authors noted that 'even if most maps characterize the global South as a space lacking in resources, members of these communities ... were able to map their communities as places that are rich in human and material resources' (p. 243). Bates et al. concluded that asset-based community mapping can allow communities to guide their own health and development rather than having solutions imposed on them by others.

Summary

Ziglio et al. (2017: 790) argue that radical change is necessary 'in order to promote health, tackle health inequities and create conditions of equity so that people can protect and promote their health'. Ziglio et al.'s observation calls for a new way of approaching the creation of health. Some of the ways that health might be created have been discussed in this chapter, including how we might create and maintain healthy public policy and what salutogenic approaches would look like. In addition, we have examined asset-based approaches to health, suggesting these as a further route to health gain. The complexities of health are mirrored in the consideration of how we might create and promote health, as reflected in the content of this chapter.

Further reading

Mittelmark, M., Bauer, G.F., Vaandrager, L., Pelikan, J.M., Sagy, S., Eriksson, M. and Lindström, C.M. (2022) *The Handbook of Salutogenesis*. 2nd edition. Springer.

This is an open-access book edited by experts on salutogenesis at the Society for Theory and Research on Salutogenesis. Drawing on theory, research, practice and policy, the book covers a large range of material and subjects, including the history of salutogenesis as an idea, Antonovsky's considerable theorizing and influence, key concepts in salutogenesis (with a comprehensive section on sense of coherence), as well as the application of salutogenic principles to a wide range of real-life settings: for example, salutogenesis and the digital world, salutogenic approaches in prisons and in healthcare settings, and salutogenic architecture.

8
Health and Our Planet

Chapter aims

- To critically consider the links between human health and planetary health
- To examine the concept of ecological health, and threats to planetary and human health
- To explore potential solutions to addressing the human and planetary health crisis

Introduction

Planetary health affects everyone. The health of our planet and our own health are intricately connected. This final chapter locates the discussion about human health in the context of planetary health. It draws attention to the critical issues of our time, including climate change, overpopulation and threats of extinction. It discusses the concept of ecological health, introducing some relevant theoretical constructs that seek to describe and explain the complex interactions between human health and the health of our planet. The chapter draws on Indigenous concepts that view human health as inextricably linked to planetary health, and discusses how both might be addressed for the benefit of all. Finally, it will consider the future of human health over the next few decades in the light of current knowledge about human and planetary health, recognizing some of the challenges that are faced and how they might be overcome.

Human and planetary health

It has long been recognized that our natural environment is important for human health (Patrick et al., 2021). As Zhang et al. (2022c: 2) argue, 'it is clear that human health is intimately related to the health of our surrounding environments, including animals and plants, and to the ecosystems on which all of us depend'. As previously discussed in this book, Indigenous perspectives have traditionally more readily embraced these connections than so-called 'western' perspectives. Whilst this has caused some significant tension and misunderstanding in the past in terms of how health is managed, maintained and promoted, we are now seeing greater appreciation (and respect) for such perspectives which locate health within a wider context, including time and place. Using the example of food, Box 8.1 illustrates how intricately everything is connected.

Climate change

We are seeing the crucial links between human health and planetary health like never before in human history. As Woodall and Cross (2022) point out, there is a general understanding that climate change is having a negative impact, not just on the planet but on human health and well-being. Climate change and associated extreme weather events impact on many dimensions of human health (Clayton, 2020), increasing the spread of infectious disease, worsening chronic disease, causing mental distress and forcing the displacement of millions of people due to drought, flooding and wildfires

Box 8.1: Food, human and planetary health (GAFF, 2022: 3 and 8)

'Food is at the heart of human, animal, and ecological health and well-being; however, our present-day food systems put all three at risk. Industrialized food systems and unhealthy diets significantly contribute to climate change, undermine the integrity of ecosystems and are responsible for the escalating rates of disease.

The effects are felt most acutely by those who are already vulnerable, including Indigenous Peoples; migrant farmers and precarious workers; people in low- or middle-income countries; and women, children, and the elderly. Broken food systems have created the ideal conditions for poor health outcomes to proliferate. Transforming the ways in which we grow, harvest, process, transport, market, consume, and dispose of food can propel us toward a more equitable, sustainable and healthy future. ...

Action at the food–health nexus will not only improve good health but is also a way to progress the climate agenda, restore valuable biodiversity, and advance social, environmental, and racial justice, all while putting forth a refreshed vision that prioritizes prevention over the curing of disease.'

– all of which is predicted to increase over the coming years (Cissé et al., 2022). 'As humans place greater pressure on the Earth's ecosystems, environmental change results in events ranging from those which are chronic, such as decreasing air quality, to [those that are] immediate, such as flooding and fires' (Smith and Nersesian, 2024: 241). Climate change is a fundamental threat to human health (Marmot, 2010). It is often referred to as a 'wicked' problem, this being 'the term used to describe some of the more challenging and complex issues of our time, many of which threaten human health' (Walls, 2018: 1). It is therefore very difficult to address on a global scale given that there are so many social, political and cultural differences between different regions of the world (Sun and Yang, 2016). Arguably climate change is the wickedest problem of all (Woodall and Cross, 2022).

Since climate change particularly affects those that are less well off and most deprived (Marmot et al., 2020), it only exacerbates existing health inequalities. The impact of it is not equally felt: some people suffer disproportionately more than others, particularly those living in low- and middle-income countries (Chancel et al., 2023; Middleton, 2022). As Chancel et al. (2023: 4) point out, 'vulnerability to numerous climate impacts is strongly linked to income and wealth, not just between countries but also within them'. For example, extreme high temperatures affect parts of the world where many people work outdoors, such as India and other parts of South Asia. In such places there are fewer opportunities to escape from the heat, and inadequate healthcare services become easily overwhelmed in heat-related emergencies. In addition, 'extreme heat not only damages agricultural yields and leads to supply drops and food insecurity in the long-term but also affects people's short-term ability to generate income from labour and purchase food' (Kroeger and Reeves, 2022: 521). Poverty therefore exacerbates the impacts of climate change and vice versa. The unprecedented heatwave in India in the first half of 2022 highlighted the vulnerability of food availability, not just in India but beyond. As Kroeger and Reeves (2022: 251) note, 'India's move to ban wheat exports amid a record-breaking heat wave show[ed] how local climate events may send shockwaves through global food security.' A final, important point to consider here is that it is the wealthier countries that produce the highest levels of greenhouse gas emissions contributing to the climate crisis: 'the global top 10% are responsible for almost half of global carbon emissions' (Chancel et al., 2023: 9). See Box 8.2 for further detail about some of the impacts of climate change.

In response to climate change, climate anxiety (or eco-anxiety) is becoming a substantial psychological burden for people across the planet (Whitmarsh et al., 2022). Whilst it is a rational response to be anxious about climate change, some people are experiencing significant harm to their mental health such that their levels of anxiety and distress interfere with their everyday lives. As Clayton (2020) points out, it is important to make a distinction between adaptive

---

Box 8.2: The impact of climate change (Chancel et al., 2023: 5)

'Climate change contributes to economic and material deprivation in myriad ways, now well documented. It aggravates low agricultural productivity in poorer countries, as well as water scarcity and security. Heat waves have significant impacts on mortality, particularly in vulnerable urban centres. Tropical cyclones and floods will continue to displace millions of people, mostly in low-income countries, and rising sea levels will make large swathes of coastal land uninhabitable. While such events will affect regions as a whole, studies point to a strong socioeconomic relationship between exposure (and especially vulnerability) and current living conditions, whereby the worst off are more affected than the rest.'

---

and maladaptive levels of climate anxiety. Adaptive anxiety provokes a meaningful response whereby a person can feel that they are able to do something to make a difference, and thereby feel more in control. It can also motivate environmental activism (Whitmarsh et al., 2022). On the other hand, maladaptive responses occur when the anxiety is so great it leads to significant disruption for the individual concerned and the inability to function as normal.

Crandon et al. (2022: 123) point out that children and young people are 'uniquely predisposed to climate anxiety' and are 'particularly vulnerable to the impacts of climate change'. A global survey on climate anxiety in 10,000 children and young people aged 16–25 in ten countries (Australia, Brazil, Finland, France, India, Nigeria, Philippines, Portugal, the UK and the US) found that children and young people in all ten countries were concerned about climate change (Hickman et al., 2021). More than half of those surveyed reported experiencing negative emotions such as sadness, anger, helplessness, guilt and worry, and more than three-quarters reported that they thought the future was frightening. When asked for their opinions about governmental responses to climate change, participants reported 'greater feelings of betrayal than of reassurance [and perceptions of] inadequate government response' (Hickman et al., 2021: e870). Not surprisingly, participants from poorer countries (i.e. India and the Philippines) – where the most extreme impacts of climate change have been experienced – had the highest levels of anxiety. However, although it can be appreciated that children and young people are more vulnerable to the long-term impact of climate change by virtue of the threat to their futures, and that they experience greater levels of climate anxiety (Whitmarsh et al., 2022), it is not just the younger generation who are suffering. The average age of adult participants in a UK study on climate anxiety by Whitmarsh et al. (2022) was 47.1 years (age range 18–85). Nearly half of the participants in this study reported that they were extremely or very worried about climate change. But the study also showed that experiencing climate anxiety can act as a catalyst for pro-environmental action and be a motivating force for making behavioural changes. See Box 8.3 for some examples of such individual behaviour changes.

Box 8.3: Individual-level actions to fight climate change by cutting carbon emissions (listed from most effective to least effective) (Wynes and Nicholas, 2017)

- Have one fewer child (or none)
- Live car-free
- Avoid flying
- Buy green energy
- Switch from electric car to car-free
- Eat a plant-based diet
- Replace typical car with hybrid
- Wash clothes in cold water
- Hang-dry clothes
- Recycle
- Upgrade light bulbs

Box 8.3 details, in order of impact, some of the actions that can be taken at an individual level to reduce carbon emissions. The most impactful action by far is to have one fewer child. Having one fewer child in a developed country is estimated to save the equivalent of 58.6 tonnes of carbon dioxide per year, as compared with the next most impactful action, living car-free, which saves approximately 2.4 tonnes per year (Wynes and Nicholas, 2017). Living car-free, avoiding long flights and eating a vegetarian diet are far more effective than other 'common green activities such as recycling, using low energy light bulbs or drying washing on a line' (Carrington, 2017: npn). Of course, we are not just talking about climate change but about environmental crisis on a much larger scale. This includes 'soil erosion, deforestation, water salinization, the systematic effects of insecticides and pesticides, toxic chemical waste, species loss, acidification of the oceans, decline of fish stocks, hormone discharges into the water supply and a multitude of other forms of devastation' (Wilkinson and Pickett, 2018: 221). The next section of this chapter discusses all this in the context of extinction threat.

Extinction threat

There is quite a lot of scientific evidence that a mass extinction event is underway. Referred to as the 'sixth mass extinction', it concerns the loss of species and the reduction of biodiversity as a result of human activity on our planet (Cafaro, 2015: 387). It is predicted that approximately 75 per cent of the Earth's species will be lost as a consequence of this (Briggs, 2017). The causes of the previous five mass extinction events in the history of the Earth were dramatic natural phenomena such as asteroid impact and volcanic activity (Cowie et al., 2022; Hernon, 2022). But the primary cause of the sixth extinction is us (Cafaro, 2015). There is a lack of agreement about the rate at which this is happening, but there is general consensus that it *is* happening. Biodiversity loss is occurring due to habitat loss, the impacts of alien species, over-exploitation (of the natural environment), pollution and climate change (Cafaro, 2015). Human activity is the root cause of all of this. Some, however, have argued that 'the world's greatest conservation problem is not species extinction, but population decline to the point where many species exist only as remnants of their former abundance' (Briggs, 2017: 234). In addition, 'there are those who do not deny an extinction crisis but accept it as a new trajectory of evolution, because humans are part of the natural world; some even embrace it, with a desire to manipulate it for human benefit' (Cowie et al., 2022: 640). Briggs (2017), for example, argues that biodiversity gains are actually taking place alongside biodiversity losses, and that some claims about the latter have been overstated in order to grab attention. The one population that is increasing, of course, is humans. The global population reached 8 billion in November 2022, an increase of approximately 6.5 billion since 1950 (United Nations, 2022). The evidence for the impact of humans on the planet is undeniable and, many contend, further impact is inevitable (Hernon, 2022; Maheshwari, 2020). Hernon (2022) argues that we do have the possibility of exercising some control over what is happening, given that is it caused by us, but that action needs to happen immediately.

Ecological health

In considering solutions to the complex challenges that have been raised so far it is useful to think about the concept of ecological health. Ecological health concerns the health of our ecosystems and the relationships between them and human health. The importance of this was starkly illustrated by the COVID-19 pandemic, where the virus passed from bats to humans and then rapidly spread around the world (Morand, 2022). Ecological health is closely related to the broader concept of planetary health. In Chapter 4 we looked at Dahlgren and Whitehead's (1991) classic 'rainbow' model of health determinants. Before we return to this, please take some time to do Pause for Reflection 8.1.

Pause for Reflection 8.1

Dahlgren and Whitehead's (1991) model of health determinants is now over thirty years old. The world has changed significantly since it was first introduced. Consider what would make it more complete? More appropriate to this point in history? Is there anything that needs to be amended? Anything that needs to be added?

Having carried out Pause for Reflection 8.1 you should be able to appreciate that the determinants of health are much more complex than they were when the rainbow model was created. In fact, several years ago, the model was further developed by Barton and Grant (2006) to include more detail. This new version of the model is known as Barton and Grant's 'health map' (see Figure 8.1).

The health map was specifically developed to take into account health determinants in relation to the built environment; however, as you can see, it includes several factors alongside those that were originally represented in the rainbow model. It is also inspired by the principle of sustainable development and by ecosystem theories (Barton

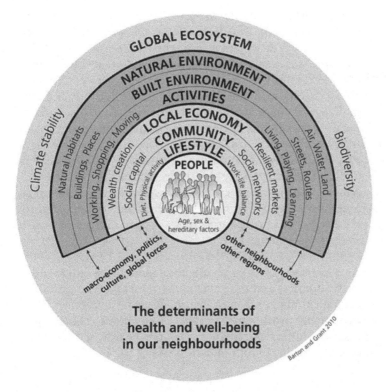

Figure 8.1 Barton and Grant's health map
Source: Barton and Grant (2006)

et al., 1995). The map includes the global ecosystem, factors such as climate stability and biodiversity, and the natural environment (natural habitats, air, water and land). Barton and Grant (2006: 252) argued that 'the environment in which we live is a major determinant of health and well-being'. Consider the health map for a moment. From a planetary perspective, do you think there is anything else missing from this representation of the determinants of health? The map considers the impact of many different things on human health, but it does not explicitly consider the impact of humans on planetary health. Nevertheless, it does illustrate the importance of ecosystems for health and is a useful tool to guide policy, planning and practice. As Barton and Grant (2006: 253) themselves suggest:

> the importance of the model is that it can be used to analyse knock-on (indirect) effects, which are often much more significant in terms of health. Take a new road, for example: the pattern of human activity – travel behaviour and destinations – is changed. Activity, in turn, affects the local natural environment (air pollution) and the global ecosystem (greenhouse emissions). It also affects local economic efficiency and people's lifestyle choices (the likelihood of walking or driving). Lifestyle changes may well affect the pattern of social networks. It is apparent that every sphere representing health determinants – except the inherited characteristics – is affected to a certain extent. The model can be used to help identify these processes and contribute to sustainability and health impact assessment.

As illustrated by the health map model, the interactions between humans and the environment are taken into account in ecological approaches to health. Without exception, local environments are bound up with our planet's ecosystems – our actions affect our planet, and the health of the planet affects our health (Smith and Nersesian, 2024).

The future of human health

We are living in what is referred to as the 'Anthropocene' geological time period: 'a new geological epoch demarcated as the time when human activities began to have a substantial global effect on the Earth's systems' (Whitmee et al., 2015: 1975). The world is witnessing ecosystem change on an unprecedented scale resulting in disasters associated with human activity on the planet (Smith and Nersesian, 2024). We are now able to appreciate that all environmental disasters are contributed to (or worsened) by human action (UNDRR, 2022). The question is, then, what can be done about it? There are many potential solutions. We have already considered some of the changes that can be made at an individual level; however, only a relatively privileged few have the means to make such changes. Change needs to happen at a higher level and must include structural, systemic solutions involving long-term policy change (Hernon, 2022). One such approach is the One Health concept, which 'addresses human, animal, and ecosystem health by fostering cooperation between several actors and stakeholders' (GAFF, 2022: 42). The One Health approach is seen as 'one of the best solutions to achieve optimal health and well-being outcomes' (Zhang et al., 2022c: 3). Zhang et al. (2022c: 4) argue that 'a One Health approach is required to tackle climate change by implementing a united, holistic action and a shift from crisis response to prevention'. See Box 8.4 for further details.

For this approach to work cooperation between many different sectors is necessary. This includes governments, researchers and workers at all levels (local, national, regional and global). It also requires information to be shared so that solutions can be found to tackle root causes and establish the connection between risks and effects (WHO, 2017). The role of communities in the One Health approach is likewise crucial. As the Centers for Disease Control and Prevention (2022) points out, the One Health concept is not new, but it has become more important in recent years, particularly in light of the COVID-19 pandemic and the threats to biodiversity. The CDCP (2022: npn) state that this is for the following reasons:

Human populations are growing and expanding into new geographical areas. As a result, more people live in close contact with wild and domestic animals, both livestock and pets. Animals play an important role in our lives, whether for food, fiber, livelihoods, travel, sport, education, or companionship. Close contact with animals and their environments provides more opportunities for disease to pass between animals and people.

The earth has experienced changes in climate and land use, such as deforestation and intensive farming practices. Disruptions in environmental conditions and habitats can provide new opportunities for diseases to pass to animals.

The movement of people, animals, and animal products has increased from international travel and trade. As a result, diseases can spread quickly across borders and around the globe.

Box 8.4: What is 'One Health'? (WHO, 2017: npn)

The World Health Organization defines 'One Health' as 'an integrated, unifying approach to balance and optimize the health of people, animals and the environment'. The One Health approach 'mobilizes multiple sectors, disciplines and communities at varying levels of society to work together. This way, new and better ideas are developed that address root causes and create long-term, sustainable solutions.'

'One Health involves the public health, veterinary and environmental sectors. The One Health approach is particularly relevant for food and water safety, nutrition, the control of zoonoses (diseases that can spread between animals and humans, such as flu, rabies and Rift Valley fever), pollution management, and combatting antimicrobial resistance (the emergence of microbes that are resistant to antibiotic therapy).'

One Health issues occurring at the human–animal–environment interface are many and complex (CDCP, 2022). Case Study 8 provides a detailed exploration of the application of the One Health approach in the Ugandan context.

Case Study 8: A One Health approach benefiting the health of people and gorillas in Uganda (adapted from GAFF, 2022: 41–5)

Uganda is home to almost half of the world's remaining mountain gorillas. Over 400 gorillas live in the rainforests of Bwindi Impenetrable National Park (BINP). Mountain gorillas are an endangered species, although their numbers have increased in recent years. This is due, in part, to the work of the non-governmental organization Conservation Through Public Health (CTPH), founded in 2003 by Dr Gladys Kalema-Zikusoka. The organization was set up after Kalema-Zikusoka found a link between an outbreak of scabies in the BINP gorillas and nearby villages that had lack of access to basic sanitation and healthcare. When the mountain gorillas sought food in the village fields they contracted scabies. Kalema-Zikusoka realized that she needed to start caring for people in order to protect the gorillas, rather than just focusing on the gorillas themselves.

Around the same time, gorilla tourism was on the increase, which led to calls for conservation. However, the villagers living on the borders of the BINP were suffering from gorillas destroying their crops. This was a significant concern given the community's reliance on subsistence farming to feed their families and to provide a small income, particularly because this is a region where hunger and malnutrition are not uncommon. The affected communities were not compensated by the tourism industry for their losses, which compounded the issue.

Kalema-Zikusoka encapsulated the solution as follows: 'everything is interlinked and interconnected. When you improve the health of humans you can improve the health of animals. When you improve the health of animals, you can also improve the health of humans.' Since 2007, CTPH, taking a multidisciplinary approach, has worked with village health teams, public health professionals, environmentalists and local communities to improve sanitation and hygiene practices and promote sustainable agriculture, among other things. There have been several outcomes. For example, community members have been supported to pursue alternative livelihoods that are not reliant on the forest for food and fuel, and tourists can buy food and crafts from the local communities.

The COVID-19 pandemic hit gorilla tourism very hard, and the communities also suffered, having no choice but to return to previous behaviours in order to survive. Poaching increased again. Whilst gorillas tend not to be poached themselves, they often fall foul of animal traps meant for other wildlife such as bush pigs, leading to injury or death. In the absence of tourism, CTPH prioritized food and farming initiatives to provide income and reduce food insecurity. This then reduced the need for the villagers to poach and minimized contact between the gorillas and the communities – to the benefit of both human and animal health.

A social enterprise project which began in 2015 engaged 500 farmers living on the edges of BINP to train them in coffee growing. There is a huge global demand for coffee, and gorillas do not like to eat coffee plants. The scheme particularly focused on women coffee farmers, promoting economic empowerment and challenging existing power dynamics. Selling coffee for export provided a revenue stream for the communities during the COVID-19 pandemic. Another related scheme provided village households with low-maintenance, fast-growing seedling crops. To prevent the gorillas from eating the crops, CTPH trained over 100 members of the communities to herd gorillas from village gardens back into the national park. 'By reducing hunger, CTPH simultaneously reduced pressure on mountain gorillas since people are now less likely to venture into the forest in search of food.' In 2021, after receiving a Champions of the Earth award, Kalema-Zikusoka was quoted as saying 'over time, the diseases that gorillas are being exposed to are reducing. It shows that when we engage communities meaningfully you can have a recovery of a population, and I'm very proud of that.'

Almost four decades ago, the Ottawa Charter for Health Promotion (WHO, 1986) identified a stable ecosystem and sustainable resources as being among the prerequisites for health. The other prerequisites referred to in the charter include social justice, equity, peace, shelter, education, food and income. Clearly, as Woodall and Cross (2022) argue, climate change disrupts many of these prerequisites, making health much more difficult to achieve. Climate change is caused by a combination of factors, some of which are natural (e.g. volcanic eruptions, solar radiation), but most of which are exacerbated by human activity and the pursuit of economic growth (use of fossil fuels, reduction in forested land), resulting in the increased greenhouse gases that are causing our world to heat up (Turrentine, 2022). Sustainability and sustainable development have been key themes in the World Health Organization's health promotion agenda for decades. As such, Baldwin (2020) argues that human and planetary health should be prioritized in policy-making. Hancock et al. (2017), among others, argue that the planet should be seen as a key setting for health promotion and that action should be taken to ensure it is taken care of in order to reduce the impact of climate change. This would be achieved by the application of the 'one planet principles'. See Box 8.5 for further details on these.

Zhang et al. (2022c) suggest that adapting to our changing climates and trying to protect people, animals and our world from the negative impacts of climate change are as important as trying to slow down the effects of climate change and mitigate for the future. As detailed in Chapter 5, the Geneva Charter for Well-being 'underlines the urgency of creating sustainable "well-being societies", committed to achieving equitable health now and for future generations without

Box 8.5: One planet principles (from Hancock et al., 2017)

Health and happiness
Encourage active, social, meaningful lives to promote good health and well-being

Equity and local economy
Create safe, equitable places to live and work, which support local prosperity and international fair trade

Culture and community
Nurture local identity and heritage, empowering communities and promoting a culture of sustainable living

Land and nature
Protect and restore land for the benefit of people and wildlife

Sustainable water
Use water efficiently, protecting local water resources and reducing flooding and drought

Local and sustainable food
Promote sustainable humane farming and healthy diets high in local, seasonal organic food and vegetable protein

Travel and transport
Reduce the need to travel and encourage walking, cycling and low-carbon transport

Materials and products
Use materials from sustainable sources and promote products and services that help people reduce consumption

Zero waste
Reduce consumption, and reuse and recycle to achieve zero waste and zero pollution

Zero carbon energy
Make buildings and manufacturing energy-efficient and supply all energy with renewables

breaching ecological limits' (WHO, 2021: 2). Greater equality is also an important factor for sustainability. It 'not only contributes to the well-being of entire populations, but also eases the path to sustainability by lessening the environmental impact of those populations' (Wilkinson and Pickett, 2018: 215).

As Smith and Nersesian (2024) argue, preparing for, responding to and recovering from disasters can be influenced by governmental responses at local, national, regional and global levels. Some disasters, especially those that reoccur, are easy to predict. Policy-makers therefore need to use foresight to address the implications and impact of climate change. Planetary health is a complex global issue that requires action across national borders (Zhang et al., 2022c). International coordination and cooperation are needed to address such issues. We are living at a critical time, witnessing the links between human and planetary health like never before. Political will is required at micro, macro and meso levels in order to make a significant and sustainable difference. The Sustainable Development Goals (SDGs) are a universal set of indicators that UN member states are now using to frame country-level policies and practices that address the critical issues of our time, including threats to human and planetary health (Warwick-Booth and Cross, 2018). See Box 8.6 for further details on the seventeen SDGs and example targets for each goal more specifically related to the issues discussed within this chapter.

Policy at all levels is crucial to tackling the urgent issues of our time. For example, policy to mitigate climate change includes encouraging active travel, provision of green and blue spaces and increasing the energy efficiency of housing (Marmot et al., 2020). The issues we have discussed in this chapter in relation to human and planetary health are complex and challenging. The advancement of the SDG agenda will contribute to addressing these issues and is an example of a global response. The Geneva Charter for Well-being (WHO, 2021) also highlights the kind of responses that are needed to address complex and interrelated global crises such as climate change. The charter states that these responses 'require investments that integrate planetary, societal, community and individual health and well-being, as well as changes in

Box 8.6: The Sustainable Development Goals

1. *End poverty in all its forms everywhere*
Associated target: by 2030, build resilience of the poor and those in vulnerable situations and reduce their exposure and vulnerability to climate-related extreme events and other economic, social and environmental shocks and disasters.

2. *End hunger, achieve food security and improved nutrition, and promote sustainable agriculture*
Associated target: by 2030, maintain the genetic diversity of seeds, cultivated plants and farmed and domesticated animals and their related wild species, including through soundly managed and diversified seed and plant banks at the national, regional and international levels, and promote access to and fair and equitable sharing of benefits arising from the utilization of genetic resources and associated traditional knowledge, as internationally agreed.

3. *Ensure healthy lives and promote well-being for all at all ages*
Associated target: by 2030, substantially reduce the number of deaths and illnesses from hazardous chemicals and air, water and soil pollution and contamination.

4. *Ensure inclusive and equitable quality education and promote lifelong learning opportunities for all*
Associated target: by 2030, eliminate gender disparities in education and ensure equal access to all levels of education and vocational training for the vulnerable, including persons with disabilities, Indigenous peoples and children in vulnerable situations.

5. *Achieve gender equality and empower all girls and women*
Associated target: undertake reforms to give women equal rights to economic resources, as well as access

to ownership and control over land and other forms of property, financial services, inheritance and natural resources, in accordance with national laws.

6. *Ensure availability and sustainable management of water and sanitation for all*
Associated target: by 2030, improve water quality by reducing pollution, eliminating dumping and minimizing release of hazardous chemicals and materials, halving the proportion of untreated wastewater and substantially increasing recycling and safe reuse globally.

7. *Ensure access to affordable, reliable, sustainable and modern energy for all*
Associated target: by 2030, increase substantially the share of renewable energy in the global energy mix.

8. *Promote sustained, inclusive and sustainable economic growth, full and productive employment and decent work for all*
Associated target: by 2030, devise and implement policies to promote sustainable tourism that creates jobs and promotes local culture and products.

9. *Build resilient infrastructure, promote inclusive and sustainable industrialization, and foster innovation*
Associated target: facilitate sustainable and resilient infrastructure development in developing countries through enhanced financial, technological and technical support to African countries, least developed countries, landlocked developing countries and small island developing States.

10. *Reduce inequality within and among countries*
Associated target: by 2030, empower and promote the social, economic and political inclusion of all irrespective of age, sex, disability, race, ethnicity, origin, religion or economic or other status.

11. *Make cities and human settlements inclusive, safe, resilient and sustainable*
Associated target: by 2030, strengthen efforts to protect and safeguard the world's cultural and natural heritage.

12. *Ensure sustainable consumption and production patterns*
Associated target: by 2030, substantially reduce waste generation through prevention, reduction, recycling and reuse.

13. *Take urgent action to combat climate change and its impacts*
Associated target: by 2030, strengthen resilience and adaptive capacity to climate-related hazards and natural disasters in all countries.

14. *Conserve and sustainably use the oceans, seas and marine resources for sustainable development*
Associated target: minimize and address the impacts of ocean acidification, including through enhanced scientific cooperation at all levels.

15. *Protect, restore and promote sustainable use of terrestrial ecosystems, sustainably manage forests, combat desertification and halt and reverse land degradation, and halt biodiversity loss*
Associated target: take urgent and significant action to reduce the degradation of natural habitats, halt the loss of biodiversity, and protect and prevent the extinction of threatened species.

16. *Promote peaceful and inclusive societies for sustainable development, provide access to justice for all and build effective, accountable and inclusive institutions at all levels*
Associated target: ensure responsive, inclusive, participatory and representative decision-making at all levels.

17. *Strengthen the means of implementation and revitalize the global partnership for sustainable development*

Associated target: promote the development, transfer, dissemination and diffusion of environmentally sound technologies to developing countries on favourable terms, including on concessional and preferential terms, as mutually agreed.

Source: https://sustainabledevelopment.un.org/focussdgs .html

social structures to support people to take control of their lives and health. Fundamental redirection of societal values and action consistent with the 2030 Agenda for Sustainable Development are required' (WHO, 2021: 2).

Finally, the Happy Planet Index is based on the premise that 'being happy is good for everyone and that promoting human happiness does not need to be at odds with creating a sustainable future'. Please take some time out to do Pause for Reflection 8.2.

Pause for Reflection 8.2

The Happy Planet Index (HPI) encourages everyone to create their own life that 'doesn't cost the earth'. You might want to do the personal HPI test provided free online at https://happyplanetindex.org/personal-hpi -test. The test will ask you several questions related to well-being, health and the environment, and then send you a personalized report giving an assessment of your happiness, health and environmental impact.

Summary

This chapter has discussed the inextricable links between human health and planetary health. Although it is not possible to do justice to these issues in one chapter, we have considered the impact of humans on the planet's health and vice versa. We have seen that ecological approaches to health are the best fit for understanding and appreciating how human and planetary health interact with each other, and for identifying where action needs to be taken to bring about change. We have considered the issues of climate change and extinction threat in some detail, noting some potential ways of tackling these, including international and local approaches to making a positive difference. The discussion has considered several such approaches, including One Health, the one planet principles and the Sustainable Development Agenda.

Further reading

Haines, A. and Frumkin, H. (2021) *Planetary Health: Safeguarding Human Health and the Environment in the Anthropocene.* Cambridge, Cambridge University Press.

This is a comprehensive textbook covering many issues pertinent to human and planetary health, including climate change, pollution, land use, biodiversity, adaptation and resilience, energy and industry, food systems and the role of health professionals in planetary health. As well as exploring how we got to where we are now, the book discusses what is required for a more sustainable future, better health and a healthier planet. It is a solution-focused approach to the issues at hand, laying out the case for transformative, cross-sectoral action. 'It presents the evidence, builds hope in our common future, and aims to motivate action by everyone … from the general public to policymakers to health professionals.'

Final Thoughts

It should be apparent by now that the answer to the question 'What is health?' is not a straightforward one. It is therefore impossible to provide a definition that will satisfy everyone. There are no easy, simple responses, as the discussion in this book has demonstrated. Perhaps the conclusion, as I have argued previously in relation to nursing practice, is that 'health is what the person says it is' (Cross, 2020). This reflects the subjective nature of health and takes into account personal perspectives and experience. However, having a collective view of health can also be beneficial, and, as we have seen, several common themes can be identified within ideas about health.

The themes that recur throughout this book include the importance of lay perspectives and the vital contribution of Indigenous concepts of health, recognition of myriad influences on ideas about health, the importance of the social determinants of health, health as a holistic notion, the value of the social model of health, the need to acknowledge and address health inequalities and inequities, the creation of health, and, finally, the inextricable links between human and planetary health.

Hopefully the contents of the book, whilst not providing a definitive answer to the question posed in its title, will have enabled you to think about health in more depth, and will have challenged any existing assumptions about the nature of health.

In conclusion, you might be thinking *why* we need to consider what health is. This is a valid question. From a health promotion perspective, which is the area I work and research in, I would always argue that we need to understand what health is in order to get alongside people to promote and improve it. Each of us brings a unique set of experiences and understandings to this issue. I anticipate that ideas about health will continue to evolve, especially in response to the changing world around us. Hopefully the discussion here has encouraged you to think about your own ideas of health, and enabled you to better understand and appreciate other peoples' perspectives on health. This might then have an impact on your own practice in the field you work in and on the people you work with.

References

Adams, C., Harder, B.M., Chatterjee, A. and Mathias, L.H. (2019) Healthworlds, cultural health toolkits, and choice: how acculturation affects patients' views of prescription drugs and prescription drug advertising. *Qualitative Health Research,* 29 (10), 1419–32.

Aggleton, P. (1990) *Health.* London, Routledge.

Alcalde-Rubio, L., Hernández-Aguado, I., Parker, L.A., Bueno-Vergara, E. and Chilet-Rosell, E. (2020) Gender disparities in clinical practice: are there any solutions? Scoping review of interventions to overcome or reduce gender bias in clinical practice. *International Journal for Equity in Health,* 19 (166), doi:10.1186/s12939-020-01283-4

Alqarni, M. (2020) Mock impoliteness in Saudi Arabia: evil eye expressive and responsive strategies. *Journal of Pragmatics,* 167, 4–19.

Angner, E. Midge, N.R., Saag, K.G. et al. (2009) Health and happiness among older adults: a community-based study. *Journal of Health Psychology,* 14 (4), 503–12.

Antonovsky, A. (1984) The Sense of Coherence as a Determinant of Health. In Matarazzo, J.D., Weiss, S.M., Herd, J.A., Miller, N.E. and Weiss, S.M. (eds.), *Behavioral Health: A Handbook of Health Enhancement and Disease Prevention.* New York, John Wiley.

Antonovsky, A. (1996) The salutogenic model as a theory to guide health promotion. *Health Promotion International,* 11, 11–18.

Arias, D., Saxena, S. and Verguet, S. (2022) Quantifying the global burden of mental disorders and their economic value. *eClinical-Medicine,* 54, doi:10.1016/jeclinm.2022.101675

Arnoldi, J. (2009) *Risk.* Cambridge, Polity Press.

Astbury, J., Schafheutle, E., Brown, J. and Cutts, C. (2021) The current and potential role of community pharmacy in asset-based approaches to health and wellbeing: a qualitative study. *International Journal of Clinical Pharmacy,* 43, 1257–64.

Atkinson, S., Bagnall, A., Cororan, R., South, J. and Curtis, S. (2019) Being well together: individual subjective and community wellbeing. *Journal of Happiness Studies,* doi:10.1007/s10902 -019-00146-2

Ayo, N. (2012) Understanding health promotion in a neoliberal climate and the making of health-conscious citizens. *Critical Public Health,* 22, 99–105.

Bache, I. (2019) How does evidence matter? Understanding 'what works' for wellbeing. *Social Indicators Research,* 142, 1153–73.

Bagnall, A. (2023) *Places, Spaces and Social Relations.* Leeds Beckett School of Health Centre for Health Promotion Research Blog,   https://www.leedsbeckett.ac.uk/blogs/school-of-health /2023/02/places-spaces-and-social-relations

Baker, S.A. and Rojeck, C. (2019) The scandal that should force us to reconsider wellness advice from influencers. *The Conversation,* https://theconversation.com/the-scandal-that-should-force-us-to -reconsider-wellness-advice-from-influencers-117041

Baldwin, L. (2020) Sustaining the Practice of Health Promotion. In Fleming, M. and Baldwin, L. (eds.) *Health Promotion in the 21st Century: New Approaches to Achieving Health for All.* London, Allen & Unwin.

Bambra, C., Fox, D. and Scott-Samuel, A. (2005) Towards a politics of health. *Health Promotion International,* 20 (2), 187–93.

Barnard, A. and Furtak, A. (2020) Psychological resilience of volunteers in a South African health care context: a salutogenic approach and hermeneutic phenomenological inquiry. *Int J Environ Res Public Health,* 17 (8), doi:10.3390/ijerph17082922

Barney, T. (2009) Power lines: the rhetoric of maps as social change in the post-Cold War Landscape. *Quarterly Journal of Speech,* 95, 412–34.

Barton, H., Davis, G. and Guise, R. (1995) *Sustainable Settlements: A Guide for Planners.* Bristol, LGMB and UWE.

Barton, H. and Grant, M. (2006) A health map for the local human habitat. *Journal of the Royal Society for the Promotion of Health,* 126 (6), 252–61.

Bates, B.R., Marvel, D.L., Nieto-Sanchez, C. and Grijalva, M.J. (2019) Community cartography in health communication:

an asset-based mapping approach in four communities in rural Ecuador. *Journal of International and Intercultural Communication,* 12 (3), 228–47.

Bauer, G.F., Roy, M., Bakibinga, P., Contu, P., Downe, S., Eriksson, M. et al. (2020) Future directions for the concept of salutogenesis: a position article. *Health Promotion International,* 35, 187–95.

BBC News (2015) Pharrell Williams addresses UN on happiness, http://www.bbc.co.uk/news/world-31997779

Beida, A., Hirschfeld, G., Schönfeld, P., Brailovskaia, J., Zhang, X.C. and Margraf, J. (2017) Universal happiness? Cross-cultural measurement invariance of scales assessing positive mental health. *Psychological Assessment,* 29 (4), 408–21.

Bell, N. (2016) Teaching by the Medicine Wheel: an Anishinaabe framework for Indigenous education. *Education Canada,* 56 (3), 1–6.

Bhatt, M. (2020) Training of the spiritual dimension of health in India: an innovative 'thought model' approach. *European Journal of Public Health,* 30 (S5), v966.

Bhattacharya, S., Pradhan, K.B., Bashar, M.A., Tripathi, S., Thiyagarajan, A. Srivastava, A. and Singh, A. (2020) Salutogenesis: a bona fide guide towards health preservation. *Journal of Family Medicine and Primary Care,* 9 (1), 16–19.

Bhattacharyya, S., Burman, R.R. and Paul, S. (2019) The concept of measuring happiness and how India can go the Nordic Way. *Critical Science,* 116 (1), 26–8.

Bishop, F. and Yardley, L. (2010) The development and initial validation of a new measure of lay definitions of health: the wellness beliefs scale. *Psychology and Health,* 25, 271–87.

Blaxter, M. (2010) *Health.* 2nd edition. Cambridge, Polity.

Bozdağ, F. and Ergün, N. (2021) Psychological resilience of healthcare professionals during COVID-19 pandemic. *Mental & Physical Health,* 124 (6), 2567–86.

Bozzola, E., Spina, G., Agostiniani, R., Barni, S., Russo, R., Scarpato, E. et al. (2022) The use of social media in children and adolescents: scoping review on the potential risks. *Int J Environ Res Public Health,* 19 (16), doi:10.3390/ijerph19169960

Brady, J., Gingras, J. and Aphramor, L. (2013) Theorizing health at every size as a relational-cultural endeavour. *Critical Public Health,* 23 (3), 345–55.

Braun-Lewensohn, O., Abu-Kaf, S. and Al-Said, K. (2020) Women in refugee camps: which coping resources help them to adapt? *Int J Environ Res Public Health,* 16 (20), doi:10.3390 /ijerph16203990

Braun-Lewensohn, O. and Mayer, C-H. (2020) Salutogenesis and coping: ways to overcome stress and conflict. *Int J Environ Res Public Health,* 17, doi:10.3390/ijerph17186667

Briggs, J.C. (2017) Emergence of a sixth mass extinction? *Biological Journal of the Linnean Society,* 122, 243–8.

British Medical Association (BMA) (2022) *Valuing Health: Why Prioritising Population Health Is Essential to Prosperity.* London, British Medical Association.

Buckley, R. (2020) Nature tourism and mental health: parks, happiness and causation. *Journal of Sustainable Tourism,* 28 (9), 1409–24.

Buettner, D., Nelson, T. and Veenhoven, R. (2020) Ways to greater happiness: a Delphi study. *Journal of Happiness Studies,* 21, 2789–806.

Burns, R.A. and Crisp, D.A. (2022) Prioritizing happiness has important implications for mental health, but perhaps only if you already are happy. *Applied Research in Quality of Life,* 17, 375–90.

Cafaro, P. (2015) Three ways to think about the sixth mass extinction. *Biological Conservation,* 192, 387–93.

Capone, D., Ferguson, A., Gribble, M. and Brown, J. (2018) Open defection sites, unmet sanitation needs, and potential sanitary risks in Atlanta, Georgia, 2017–2018. *American Journal of Public Health,* 108 (9), 1238–40.

Caprioli, L., Larson, M., Ek, R. and Ooi, C.-S. (2021) The inevitability of essentializing culture in destination branding: the cases of *fika* and *hygge. Journal of Place Management and Development,* 14 (3), 346–61.

Carrington, D. (2017) Want to fight climate change? Have fewer children. *The Guardian,* 12 July.

Cassetti, V., Powell, K., Barnes, A. and Sanders, T. (2019) A systematic scoping review of asset-based approaches to promote health in communities: development of a framework. *Global Health Promotion,* 27 (3), 15–23.

Cassinger, C., Lucarelli, A. and Gyimothy, S. (2019) *The Nordic Wave in Place Branding: Poetics, Practices, Politics.* Cheltenham, Edward Elgar.

CDCP (2018) *Emotional Well-Being,* https://www.cdc.gov/emotional-wellbeing/index.htm

CDCP (Centers for Disease Control and Prevention) (2022) One Health, www.cdc.gov/onehealth/basics/index.html

Chancel, L., Bothe, P. and Voituriez, T. (2023) *Climate Inequality Report 2023.* World Inequality Lab.

Charlton, A. (2004) Medicinal uses of tobacco in history. *Journal of the Royal Society of Medicine,* 97 (6), 292–6.

Chen, H.T. (2017) The contribution of mobile social media to social capital and psychological well-being: examining the role of communicative use, friending and self-disclosure. *Computers in Human Behavior,* 75, 958–65.

Cheng, Z., Prakash, K., Smyth, R. and Wang, H. (2020) Housing wealth and happiness in urban China. *Cities,* 96, doi:10.1016/j.cities.2019.102470

Chirico, F. (2016) Spiritual well-being in the 21st century: it's time to review the current WHO's health definition. *Journal of Health and Social Sciences,* 1 (1), 11–16.

Chronin de Chavez, A., Backett-Milburn, K., Parry, O. and Platt, S. (2005) Understanding and researching wellbeing: its usage in different disciplines and potential for health research and health promotion. *Health Education Journal,* 64 (1), 70–87.

Cissé, G., McLeman, R., Adams, R., Aldunce, P., Browne, K., Campbell-Lendrum, D. et al. (2022) Health, Wellbeing, and the Changing Structure of Communities. In *Climate Change 2022: Impacts, Adaptation, and Vulnerability. Contribution of Working Group II to the Sixth Assessment Report of the Intergovernmental Panel on Climate Change.* Cambridge, Cambridge University Press.

Clark, A., Fléche, S., Layard, R., Powdthavee, N. and Ward, G. (2017) *The Key Determinants of Happiness and Misery.* CEP Discussion Papers, CEDP1485. London Centre for Economic Performance, London School of Economics and Political Science.

Clayton, S. (2020) Climate anxiety: psychological responses to climate change. *Journal of Anxiety Disorders,* 74, doi:10.1016/j.janxdis.2020.102263

Cloninger, R.C. and Zohar, A.H. (2011) Personality and the perception of health and happiness. *Journal of Affective Disorders,* 128 (1–2), 24–32.

Colino, S. and Young, A. (2022) What is hygge, and why is it good for your well-being?, www.everydayhealth.com/wellness/what-is-hygge-and-why-is-it-good-for-your-wellbeing

Cowie, R.H., Bouchet, P. and Fontaine, B. (2022) The sixth mass extinction: fact, fiction or speculation? *Biological Reviews,* 97, 640–63.

Crandon, T.J., Scott, J.G., Charlson, F.J. and Thomas, H.J. (2022) A social-ecological perspective on climate anxiety in children and adolescents. *Nature Climate Change,* 12, 123–31.

Crawford, R. (2006) Health as meaningful social practice. *Health,* 10 (4), 401–20.

Cross, R. (2013) *The Social Construction of Risk: Young Women and Health.* Unpublished PhD. Leeds Beckett University.

Cross, R. (2020) Understanding the importance of concepts of health. *Nursing Standard, 35* (12), 61–5.

Cross, R., Davis, S. and O'Neil, I. (2017) *Health Communication: Theoretical and Critical Perspectives.* Cambridge, Polity.

Cross, R., Rowlands, S. and Foster, S. (2021a) The Foundations of Health Promotion. In Cross, R., Warwick-Booth, L., Rowlands, S., Woodall, J., O'Neil, I. and Foster, S. *Health Promotion: Global Principles and Practice.* 2nd edition. Wallingford, CABI.

Cross, R., Warwick-Booth, L. and Foster, S. (2021b) Towards the Future of Health Promotion. In Cross, R., Warwick-Booth, L., Rowlands, S., Woodall, J., O'Neil, I. and Foster, S. *Health Promotion: Global Principles and Practice.* 2nd edition. Wallingford, CABI.

Cross, R. and Woodall, J. (2024) *Green and Tones' Health Promotion: Planning and Strategies.* 5th edition. London, Sage.

Crossley, M. (2003) 'Would you consider yourself a healthy person?' using focus groups to explore health as a moral phenomenon. *Journal of Health Psychology,* 8, 501–14.

Cunningham, S., Hudson, C.C. and Harkness, K. (2021) Social media and depression symptoms: a meta-analysis. *Res Child Adolesc Psychopathol,* 49, 241–53.

Dahlgren, G. and Whitehead, M. (1991) *Policies and Strategies for Promoting Social Equity in Health.* Stockholm, Institute of Futures Studies.

Dahlgren, G. and Whitehead, M. (2007) *Policies and Strategies for Promoting Social Equity in Health.* Background document to WHO – Strategy Paper for Europe. Stockholm, Institute for Futures Studies.

Daniel-González, L., Moral-de le Rubia, J., Valle-de la, A., Martínez-Martí, M.L. and García-Cadena, C.H. (2023) A predictive model of happiness among medical students. *Current Psychology,* 42, 955–66.

Dapice, A.N. (2006) The Medicine Wheel. *Journal of Transcultural Nursing,* 17 (3), 251–60.

Das, K.V., Jones-Harrell, C., Fan, Y., Ramaswami, A., Orlove, B. and Botchwey, N. (2020) Understanding subjective wellbeing: perspectives from psychology and public health. *Public Health Review,* 41, doi:10.1186/s40985-020-00142-5

De Jong, N., Collins, A. and Plűg, S. (2019) 'To be healthy to me is to be free': how discourses of freedom are used to construct healthiness among young South African adults. *International Journal of Qualitative Studies on Health and Well-being,* 14, doi:10.1080/17482631.2019.1603518

Delle Fave, A., Brdar, I., Wissing, M.P., Araujo, U., Castro Solano, A., Freire, T. et al. (2016) Lay definitions of happiness across nations: the primacy of harmony and relational connectedness. *Frontiers in Psychology,* doi:10.338/fspyg.2016.00030

Detthippornpong, S., Songwathana, P. and Bourbonnais, A. (2021) '*Bai Lod*' holistic health experienced by homebound older people in the southern Thai community. *Int J Older People Nurs,* 16, doi: 10.1111/opn.12364

Detthippornpong, S., Songwathana, P and Bourbonnais, A. (2022) Holistic health practices of rural Thai homebound older adults: a focused ethnographic study. *Journal of Transcultural Nursing,* 33 (4), 521–8.

Diener, E., Heintzelman, S.J., Kushlev, K., Tay, L., Wirtz, D., Lutes, L. and Oishi, S. (2017) Findings all psychologists should know from the new science on subjective well-being. *Canadian Psychology,* 58 (2), 87–104.

Dodge, R., Daly, A.P., Huyton, J. and Sanders, L.D. (2012) The challenge of defining wellbeing. *International Journal of Wellbeing,* 2 (3), 222–35.

Dolan, P. (2019) *Happy Ever After: Escaping the Myth of the Perfect Life.* London, Allen Lane.

Downey, C.A. and Chang, E.C. (2013) Assessment of everyday beliefs about health: the lay concepts of health inventory, college student version. *Psychology and Health,* 28 (7), 818–32.

Duncan, P. (2013) Failing to professionalise, struggling to specialise: the rise and fall of health promotion as a putative specialism in England, 1980–2000. *Medical History,* 57 (3), 377–96.

Dykhuizen, M., Marshall, K., Walker, R.L. and Saddleback, J. (2022) Holistic health of two-spirit people in Canada: a call for nursing action. *Journal of Holistic Nursing,* 40 (4), 383–96.

Earle, S. (2007) Exploring Health. In Earle, S., Lloyd, C.E., Sidell, M. and Spurr, S. (eds.) *Theory and Research in Promoting Public Health.* London, Sage.

Ehsan, A., Klaasm H.S., Bastianen, A. and Spini, D. (2019) Social capital and health: a systematic review of systematic reviews. *Population Health,* 8, doi:10.1016/j.ssmph.2019.100425

Eriksson, M. and Lindström, B. (2005) Validity of Antonovsky's sense of coherence scale: a systematic review. *J Epidemiol Community Health,* 59, 460–6.

Eriksson, M. and Lindström, B. (2008) A salutogenic interpretation of the Ottawa Charter. *Health Promotion International,* 23 (2), 190–9.

Evli, M. and Şimşek, N. (2022) The effect of COVID-19 uncertainty on internet addiction, happiness and life satisfaction in adolescents. *Archives of Psychiatric Nursing,* 41, 20–6.

Fallon, C.F. and Karlawish, J. (2019) Is the WHO definition of health aging well? Frameworks for 'health' after three score and ten. *American Journal of Public Health,* 109 (8), doi:10.2105/AJPH.2019.305177

Farand, C. (2017) Women spend more years of their life in poor health than men, major new report finds. *Independent,* 18 July.

Farshadnia, E., Koochakzaei, M., Borji, M., Khorrami, Z. and Memaryan, N. (2018) Spiritual health as a predictor of social and general health in university students? A study in Iran. *Pastoral Psychology,* 67, 493–504.

Felton, I. (2021) What does a healthy society look like?, www.ianfelton/com/post/what-does-a-healthy-society-look-like

Fijal, D. and Beagan, B.L. (2019) Indigenous perspectives on health: integration with a Canadian model of practice. *Canadian Journal of Occupational Therapy,* 86 (3), 220–31.

Fisher, J.W., Francis, L.J. and Johnson, P. (2000) Assessing spiritual health via four domains of spiritual wellbeing: the SH4DI. *Pastoral Psychology,* 49 (2), 133–45.

Fleming, M. and Baldwin, L. (2020) *Health Promotion in the 21st Century: New Approaches to Achieving Health for All.* London, Allen & Unwin.

Fleming, M., Parker, E. and Baldwin, L. (2020) The Changing Nature of Health Promotion. In Fleming, M. and Baldwin, L. (eds.) *Health Promotion in the 21st Century: New Approaches to Achieving Health for All.* London, Allen & Unwin.

Flood, D. and Rohloff, P. (2018) Indigenous languages and global health. *The Lancet,* 6, e134–5.

Forgeard, M.J.C., Jayawickreme, E., Kern, M.L. and Seligman, M.E.P. (2011) Doing the right thing: measuring wellbeing for public policy. *International Journal of Wellbeing,* 1 (1), 79–106.

Fortier, M.S. and Morgan, T.L. (2022) How optimism and physical activity interplay to promote happiness. *Current Psychology,* 41, 8559–67.

Freak-Poli, R., Ryan, J., Tran, T., Owen, A., McHugh Power, J., Berk, M. et al. (2022) Social isolation, social support and loneliness as independent concepts, and their relationship with health-related quality of life among older women. *Aging & Mental Health,* 26 (7), 1335–44.

Frederick, D.A., Saguy, A.C. and Gruys, K. (2016) Culture, health and bigotry: how exposure to cultural accounts of fatness shape attitudes about health risk, health policies, and weight-based prejudice. *Social Science & Medicine,* 165, 271–9.

Friedli, L. (2013) 'What we've tried, hasn't worked': the politics of assets-based public health. *Critical Public Health,* 23 (2), 131–45.

Friesen, P. (2018) Personal responsibility within health policy: unethical and ineffective. *Journal of Medical Ethics,* 44 (1), 53–8.

GAFF (Global Alliance for the Future of Food) (2022) *Creating Better Health for People, Animals, & the Planet: Food Systems Insights for Health Professionals.* Global Alliance for the Future of Food.

Germond, P. and Cochrane, J. (2010) Healthworlds: conceptualising landscapes of health & healing. *Sociology,* 44, 307–24.

Ghaderi, A., Tabatabaei, S.M., Nedjat, S., Javadi, M. and Larijani, B. (2018) Explanatory definition of the concept of spiritual health: a qualitative study in Iran. *J Med Ethics Hist Med,* 11 (3), PMC6150917.

Ghaemi, N.S. (2011) The biopsychosocial model in psychiatry: a critique. *Existenz: An International Journal in Philosophy, Religion, Politics, and the Arts,* 6 (1), 1–8.

Glasgow Centre for Population Health (2011) *Asset-Based Approaches for Health Improvement: Redressing the Balance.* Briefing Paper Concept Series 9. Glasgow Centre for Population Health.

Global Burden of Disease (GBD) (2023) About GBD, www.healthdata.org/gbd/about

Gopalkrishnan, N. (2018) Cultural diversity and mental health: considerations for policy and practice. *Frontiers in Public Health,* 6, doi:10.3389/fpubh.2018.00179

Graham, H. (2009) *Understanding Health Inequalities.* 2nd edition. Buckingham, Open University Press.

Grant, A.M., Christianson, M.K. and Price, R.H. (2007) Happiness, health, or relationships? Managerial practices and employee wellbeing trade-offs. *Academy of Management Perspectives,* 21 (3), 51–63.

Green, J., Cross, R., Woodall, J. and Tones, K. (2019) *Health Promotion: Planning and Strategies.* 4th edition. London, Sage.

Green, J., Steinbach, R. and Datta, J. (2012) The travelling citizen: emergent discourses of moral mobility in a study of cycling in London. *Sociology,* 46, 272–89.

Gregg, J. and O'Hara, L. (2007) The Red Lotus Health Promotion Model: a new model for holistic, ecological and salutogenic health promotion practice. *Health Promotion Journal of Australia,* 18, 12–19.

Gu, J., Strauss, C., Bond, R. and Cavanagh, K. (2015) How do mindfulness-based cognitive therapy and mindfulness-based reduction improve mental health and wellbeing? A systematic review and meta-analysis of mediation studies. *Clinical Psychology Review,* 37, 1–12.

Guerci, M., Hauff, S. and Gilardi, S. (2022) High-performance work practices and their associations with health, happiness and relational well-being: are there any tradeoffs? *International Journal of Human Resource Management,* 33 (2), 329–59.

Gustafson, T. (2011) The civic duty to maintain health, https:// citizenthink.wordpress.com/2011/11/30/the-civic-duty-to -maintain-health

Gyasi, R.M., Accam, B.T., Forkour, D., Marfo, C.O., Adjakloe, Y.A.D., Abass, K. et al. (2023) Emotional and physical-related experiences as potential mechanisms linking physical activity and happiness: evidence from the Ghana Aging, Health, Psychological Well-being and Health-seeking Behavior Study. *Archives of Psychiatric Nursing,* 42, 113–21.

Hallam, K.T., Bilsborough, S. and de Counten, M. (2018) 'Happy feet': evaluating the benefits of a 100-day 10,000 step challenge on mental health and wellbeing. *BCM Psychiatry,* 18 (19), doi:10.1186/s12888-018-1609-y

Hancock, T., Capon, A., Dooris, M. and Patrick, R. (2017) One planet regions: planetary health at the local level. *The Lancet Planetary Health,* 21, e92–3.

Happiness Research Institute (2020) Our research, www .happinessresearchinstitute.com/happinessresearch

Harrop, E., Addis, S., Elliott, E. and Williams, G. (2007) *Resilience, Coping and Salutogenic Approaches to Maintaining and Generating Health: A Review.* Cardiff, Cardiff Institute of Society, Health and Ethics, Cardiff University.

Hatala, A., McGavock, J., Michaelson, V. and Pickett, W. (2021) Low risks for spiritual highs: risk-taking behaviours and the protective benefits of spiritual health among Saskatchewan adolescents. *Paediatrics & Child Health,* 26 (2), doi:10.1093 /pch/pxaa007

Healthy People 2030 (2020) *Social Determinants of Health.* Office of Disease Prevention and Health Promotion, US Department of Health and Human Services, www.health.gov/healthypeople /priority-areas/social-determinants-health

Helliwell, J.F., Layard, R., Sachs, J.D., De Neve, J-E., Aknin, L.B., Wang, S. and Paculor, S. (2023) *World Happiness Report,* https://worldhappiness.report

Henriques, G. (2015) The biopsychosocial model and its limita-tions. *Psychology Today,* 30 October, www.psychologytoday .com

Hernon, N. (2022) Will climate change make a sixth mass extinction an inevitability? *Routes,* 3 (1), 33–42.

Hickman, C., Marks, E., Pihkala, P., Clayton, S., Lewandowski, R.E., Mayall, E.E. et al. (2021) Climate anxiety in children and young people and their beliefs about government responses to climate change: a global survey. *Lancet Planet Health,* 5, e863–73.

Hilkens, L., Cruyff, M., Woertman, L., Benjamins, J. and Evers, C. (2021) Social media, body image and resistance training: creating the perfect 'me' with dietary supplements, anabolic steroids and SARM's. *Sports Medicine – Open,* 7, doi:10.1186 /s40798-021-00371-1

Hills, P. and Argyle, M. (2002) The Oxford Happiness Questionnaire: a compact scale for the measurement of psychological well-being. *Personality and Individual Differences,* 33 (7), 1073–82.

Hinson, S., Bolton, P. and Kennedy, S. (2023) *Fuel Poverty in the UK. Research Briefing.* 24 March. London, House of Commons Library.

Hjelm, J.R. (2010) *Dimensions of Health: Conceptual Models.* London, Jones and Barlett.

Hofmann, B. (2019) Human enhancement: enhancing health or harnessing happiness? *Bioethical Inquiry,* 16, 87–98.

Holwerda, T.J., van Tilburg, T.G., Deeg, D.J.H., Schutter, N., Van, R., Dekker, J. et al. (2016) The impact of loneliness and depression on mortality: results from the Longitudinal Ageing Study in Amsterdam. *British Journal of Psychiatry,* 209, 127–34.

Horton, R. (2016) The secrets of a healthy society. *The Lancet,* 23 January, doi:10.1016/S0140-6736(16)00106-9

Hossain, M.M., Tasnim, S., Sultana, A., Faizah, F., Mazumder, H., Zou, L., McKyer, E.L.J., Ahmed, H.U. and Ma, P. (2020) Epidemiology of mental health problems in COVID-19: a review. *F1000Res,* 9 (636), doi:10.12688/f1000research.24457.1

Huber, M. (2011) How should we define health? *British Medical Journal,* 343 doi:10.1136/bmj.d4163

Hubley, J., Copeman, J. and Woodall, J. (2021) *Practical Health Promotion.* 3rd edition. Cambridge, Polity.

Iacobucci, G. (2021) Covid-19: England sees biggest fall in life expectancy since records began in wake of pandemic. *BMJ,* 374, doi:10.1136/bmj.n2291

Irby, M.B., Ballard, P.J., Locklear, T., Jeffries-Logan, V., Brewington, T., Byrd, R. et al. (2021) Native pathways to health: a culturally grounded and asset-based CBPR project exploring the health of

North Carolina's American Indian communities. *North Carolina Medical Journal,* 82 (6), 398–405.

Jaberi, A., Momennsab, M., Yetatalab, S., Ebadi, A. and Cheraghi, M.A. (2017) Spiritual health: a concept analysis. *Journal of Religion and Health,* doi:10.1007/s10943-017-0379-z

Javani, Z., Madani, R., Hojat, I. and Zadeh, R. (2019) The relationship between daylight and happiness for women in residential districts of Isfahan, Iran. *Environ Qual Manage,* 28, 103–10.

Jo, H.K., Kim, H.K. and Jeong, J.N. (2020) Factors affecting happiness among rural residents: a cross sectional survey. *Community Mental Health Journal,* 56, 915–24.

Johnson, C. (2007) *Creating Health for Everyone: Principles, Practice and Philosophy.* Morrisville, NC, Lulu Press.

Johnson, D., Deterding, S., Kuhn, K., Staneva, A., Stouanov, S. and Hides, S. (2016) Gamification for health and wellbeing: a systematic review of the literature. *Health Interventions,* 6, 89–106.

Kane, M., Thornton, J. and Bibby, J. (2022) *Building Public Understanding of Health and Health Inequalities.* London, The Health Foundation.

Kaptchuk, T.J. and Miller, (2015) Placebo effects in medicine. *N Engl J Med,* 373 (1), 8–9.

Karimi, M. and Brazier, J. (2016) Health, health-related quality of life, and quality of life: what is the difference? *Pharmacoeconomics,* 34 (7), 645–9.

Kawachi, I. (2010) The Relationship between Health Assets, Social Capital and Communities. In Morgan, A., Davies, M. and Ziglio, E. (eds.) *Health Assets in a Global Context.* New York, Springer.

Kelley, M.L. (2010) An Indigenous issue: why now? *Journal of Palliative Care,* 26 (1), 5.

Kelly, C., Kasperavicius, D., Duncan, D., Etherington, C., Giangregorio, L., Presseau, J. et al. (2021) 'Doing' or 'using' intersectionality? Opportunities and challenges in incorporating intersectionality into knowledge translation theory and practice. *International Journal for Equity in Health,* 20 (187), doi:10 .1186/s12939-021-01509-z

Kennedy, E., Binder, G., Humphries-Waa, K., Tidhar, T., Cini, K., Comrie-Thomson, L. et al. (2022) Gender inequalities in health and wellbeing across the first two decades of life: an analysis of 40 low-income and middle-income countries in the Asia-Pacific region. *Lancet Glob Health,* 8: e1473–88, doi:10.1016/S2214 -109X(20)30354-5

Kickbusch, I. (2012) Editorial: 21st century determinants of health and wellbeing: a new challenge for health promotion. *Global Health Promotion,* 19 (3), 1757–9.

Kiran, T. and Pinto, A.D. (2016) Swimming 'upstream' to tackle the social determinants of health. *BMJ Quality & Safety,* 25, 138–40.

Knai, C. and Savona, N. (2023) A Systems Perspective on the Pathways of Influence of Commercial Determinants of Health. In Maani, N., Petticrew, M. and Galea, S. (eds.) *The Commercial Determinants of Health.* Oxford, Oxford University Press.

Kreiger, N. (2008) Proximal, distal and the politics of causation: what's level got to do with it? *American Journal of Public Health,* 98 (2), 221–30.

Kroeger, C. and Reeves, A. (2022) Extreme heat leads to short- and long-term food insecurity with serious consequences for health. *European Journal of Public Health,* 32 (4), 521.

Kross, E., Verduyn, P., Sheppes, G., Costello, C.K., Jonides, J. and Ybarra, O. (2021) Social media and well-being: pitfalls, progress, and next steps. *Trends in Cognitive Sciences,* 25, 55–66.

Krys, K., Park, J., Kocimska-Zych, A., Kosiarczyk, A., Selim, H.A., Wojtczuk-Turek, A. et al. (2021) Personal life satisfaction as a measure of societal happiness is an individualistic presumption: evidence from fifty countries. *Journal of Happiness Studies,* 22, 2197–14.

Kumar, A. and Nayar, K.R. (2020) COVID-19 and its mental health consequences. *Journal of Mental Health,* 30 (1), doi:10.1080 /09638237.2020.1757052

Labonté, R. (1998) Health promotion and the common good: towards a politics of practice. *Critical Public Health,* 8 (2), 107–29.

Lacy-Nichols, J., de Lacy-Vawdon, C. and Moodie, R. (2023) Defining the Commercial Determinants of Health. In Maani, N., Petticrew, M. and Galea, S. (eds.) *The Commercial Determinants of Health.* Oxford, Oxford University Press.

Lalonde, M. (1974) *A New Perspective on the Health of Canadians.* Ottawa, Ministry of Health and Welfare.

The Lancet (2016) Health and happiness. Editorial, *The Lancet,* 387, 1251.

The Lancet (2020) Global health: time for radical change? *The Lancet,* 369, 1129.

The Lancet (2023) *Global Burden of Disease,* www.thelancet.com/ gdb

Lavallée, L. (2013) Balancing the Medicine Wheel through physical activity. *International Journal of Indigenous Health,* 4 (1), 64–71.

Laverack, G. (2004) *Health Promotion Practice: Power and Empowerment.* London, Sage.

Lawrence, E.M., Rogers, R.G., Zajacova, A. and Wadsworth, T. (2019) Marital happiness, marital status, health, and longevity. *Journal of Happiness Studies,* 20, 1539–61.

Layard, R. (2011) *Happiness: Lessons from a New Science.* 2nd edition. London, Penguin.

Lederman, Z. (2023) Loneliness – a clinical primer. *Br Med Bull.,* 7 Feb, doi:10.1093/bmb/ldad003

Lee, A., Sinha, I., Boyce, T., Allen, J. and Goldblatt, P. (2022) *Fuel Poverty, Cold Homes and Health Inequalities in the UK.* London, Institute of Health Equity.

Lee, B.X. (2019) *Violence: An Interdisciplinary Approach to Causes, Consequences and Cures.* London, Wiley.

Lenza, C. (2020) Eating disorders in 'millennials': risk factors and treatment strategies in the digital age. *Clinical Social Work Journal,* 48, 46–53.

Lin, W.-H., Pan, W.-C. and Yi, C.-C. (2019) 'Happiness in the air?' The effects of air pollution on adolescent happiness. *BMC Public Health,* 19 (1), doi:10.1186/s12889-019-7119-0

Lindström, B. and Eriksson, M. (2006) Contextualizing salutogenesis and Antonovsky in public health development. *Health Promotion International,* 21 (3), 5–9.

Lindström, B. and Eriksson, M. (2009) The salutogenic approach to the making of HiAP/healthy public policy: illustrated by a case study. *Global Health Promotion,* 16 (1), 17–28.

Liu, Y., Zhu, K., Li, R.-L., Song, Y. and Zhang, Z.-J. (2021) Air pollution impairs subjective happiness by damaging their health. *Int J Environ Res Public Health,* 18, doi:10.3390/ijerph181910319

Love, R., Moore, M. and Warburton, J. (2017) Nurturing spiritual well-being among older people in Australia: drawing on Indigenous and non-Indigenous ways of knowing. *Australasian Journal on Ageing,* 36, 180–6.

LSE (2016) Relationships and good health the key to happiness, https://www.lse.ac.uk/News/Latest-news-from-LSE/2016/12-December-2016-1/Relationships-and-happiness

Lucas, K. and Lloyd, B. (2005) *Health Promotion: Evidence and Experience.* London, Sage.

Lupton, D. (2012) *Medicine as Culture: Illness, Disease and the Body.* 3rd edition. London, Sage.

Lupton, D. and Peterson, A. (1996) *The New Public Health.* London, Sage.

Lyubomirsky, S. and Lepper, H. (1999) A measure of subjective happiness: preliminary reliability and construct validation. *Social Indicators Research,* 46, 137–55.

Maani, N., Petticrew, M. and Galea, S. (2023) Commercial Determinants of Health: An Introduction. In Maani, N., Petticrew, M. and Galea, S. (eds.) *The Commercial Determinants of Health.* Oxford, Oxford University Press.

McDaid, L., Hunt, K., McMillan, L., Russell, S., Milne, D., Illett, R. and Lorimer, K. (2019) Absence of holistic sexual health understandings among men and women in deprived areas of Scotland: qualitative study. *BMC Public Health,* 19, 299, doi:10.1186 /s12889-019-6558-y

McDonald, C. (2023) Problems with the WHO definition of 'health', www.catherinemcdonald.net

McIntosh, J., Marques, B. and Mwipiko, R. (2021) Therapeutic Landscapes and Indigenous Culture: Māori Health Models in Aotearoa/New Zealand. In Spee, J.C. et al. (eds.) *Clan and Tribal Perspectives on Social, Economic and Environmental Sustainability.* Emerald Publishing Limited (ebook).

Mackenbach, J.P. (2022) Omran's 'epidemiological transition' 50 years on. *International Journal of Epidemiology,* 51 (4), 1054–7.

Magnúsdóttir, I., Lovik, A. Unnarsdóttir, A.B., McCartney, D., Ask, H. and Kõiv, K. et al. (2022) Acute COVID-19 severity and mental health morbidity trajectories in patient population of six nations: an observational study. *Lancet Public Health,* 7, e406–16, doi:10.1016/S2468-2667(22)00042-1

Maheshwari, A. (2020) Extinction is inevitable in the globalized world. *Human Dimensions of Wildlife,* 26, 501–2.

Makridis, C.A. and Wu, C. (2021) How social capital helps communities weather the COVID-19 pandemic. *PLOS ONE,* 16 (9), doi:10.1371/journal.pone.0258021

Malinakova, K., Kopcakova, J., Geckova, A.M., van Dijk, J.P., Furstova, J., Kalman, M., Tavel, T. and Reijneveld, S.A. (2018) 'I am spiritual but not religious': does one without the other protect against adolescent health-risk behaviour? *International Journal of Public Health,* 64: 115–24.

Mana, A., Grossi-Milani, R., Penachiotti, F.D.F., Hardy, L.J., Canal, D.J., Benheim, S. et al. (2021) Salutogenesis in the time of COVID-19: what coping resources enable people to face crisis and stay well? International and longitudinal study. *Academia Letters,* Article 4322, doi:10.20935/AL4322

Manstead, A.S.R. (2018) The psychology of social class: how socioeconomic status impacts thoughts, feelings, and behaviour. *British Journal of Social Psychology,* 57, 267–91.

Marmot, M. (2010) *Fair Society, Healthy Lives: Strategies Review of Health Inequalities in England Post-2010.* London, Institute of Health Equity.

Marmot, M. Allen, J., Boyce, T., Goldblatt, P. and Morrison, J. (2020) *Health Equity in England: The Marmot Review 10 Years On.* London, Institute of Health Equity.

Martin, G.P. (2008) 'Ordinary people only': knowledge, representativeness, and the publics of public participations in health care. *Sociology of Health and Illness,* 30 (1), 35–54.

Meldgaard, J., Jespersen, L.N., Anderson, T.H. and Grabowski, D. (2022) Exploring protective factors through positive psychology and salutogenesis in Danish families with type 2 diabetes. *Health Promotion International,* 37, doi:10.1093/heapro/daab156

Middleton, J. (2022) President's message for July 2022 – Groundhog Day: climate emergency is with us again. *The Association of Schools of Public Health in the European Region,* https://www .aspher.org/articles,4,149.html

Miething, A., Mewes, J. and Giordano, G.N. (2020) Trust, happiness and mortality: findings from a prospective US population-based survey. *Social Science & Medicine,* 252, doi:10.1016/j.socscimed .2020.112809

Millman, E., Lee, S. and Neimeyer, R. (2020) Social isolation and the mitigation of coronavirus anxiety: the meditating role of meaning. *Journal of Death Studies,* doi:10.1080/07481187.2020 .1775362

Mitonga-Monga, J. and Mayer, C-H. (2020) Sense of coherence, burnout, and work engagement: the moderating effect of coping in the Democratic Republic of Congo. *Int J Environ Res Public Health,* 17 (11), doi:10.3390/ijerph17114127

Moeini, B., Barati, M., Farhadian, M. and Ara, M.H. (2019) The effectiveness of an educational intervention to enhance happiness in Iranian older people: applying social support theory. *Australasian Journal on Ageing,* 39 (1), e86–93.

Moksnes, U.K. and Espnes, G.A. (2020) Sense of coherence in association with stress experience and health in adolescents. *Int J Environ Res Public Health,* 17 (9), doi:10.3390/ijerph17093003

Moorley, C., Cahill, S. and Corcoran, N. (2016) Stroke among African-Caribbean women: lay beliefs of risks and causes. *Journal of Clinical Nursing,* 25, 403–11.

Morand, S. (2022) One Health: an ecosystem-based ecology of health. *Journal of Field Actions,* 24, 58–63.

Morgan, A. and Ziglio, E. (2007) Revitalising the evidence base for public health: an assets model. *Promotion & Education,* 14 (Suppl 2), 17–22.

Morilla, G.S. and del Palacio, A.E. (2016) Health from the humanist perspective of Blas Álvarez de Miraval. *Revista Internacional de Medicina y Ciencias de al Actividad Física y el Deporte*, 16 (64), 757–73.

Morrison, V. and Bennett, P. (2016) *Introduction to Health Psychology*. 4th edition. Harlow, Pearson Education.

Murray, C.J.L. (2022) The Global Burden of Disease Study at 30 years. *Nature Medicine*, 28, 2019–26.

Nadal, D., Hampson, K., Lembo, T., Rodrigues, R., Vanak, A.T. and Cleveland, S. (2022) Where rabies is not a disease: bridging healthworlds to improve mutual understanding and prevention of rabies. *Front. Vet. Sci*, 9, doi:10.3389/fvets.2022.867266

Nampewo, Z., Mike, J.H. and Wolff, J. (2022) Respecting, protecting and fulfilling the human right to health. *Int J Equity Health*, 21, doi:10.1186/s12939-022-01634-3

Nanjunda, D.C. (2015) A theoretical retrospection of changing social construction of health and illness. *Al Ameen J Med Sci*, 8 (3), 175–8.

Neilsen, T.W. and Ma, J.S. (2021) Examining the social characteristics underpinning Danish 'hygge' and their implications for promoting togetherness in multicultural education. *Multicultural Education Review*, 13 (2), doi:10.1080/2005615X.2021.1919964

Nelson, S.L., Harriger, J.A., Miller-Perrin, C. and Rouse, S.V. (2022) The effects of body-positive Instagram posts on body image in adult women. *Body Image*, 42, 338–46.

O'Hara, L., Ahmed, H. and Elashie, S. (2021) Evaluating the impact of a brief Health at Every Size®-informed health promotion activity on body positivity and internalized weight-based oppression. *Body Image*, 73, 225–37.

Olafsdottir, S. (2013) Social Construction and Health. In Cockerham, W. (ed.) *Medical Sociology on the Move*. Dordrecht, Springer.

Oleribe, O.O., Ukwedeh, O., Burstow, N.J., Gomaa, A.I., Sonderup, M.W., Cook, N. et al. (2018) Health: redefined. *Pan African Medical Journal*, 30 (292), 10.11604/pamj.2018.30.292.15436

Open Education Sociology Dictionary (2023) Structure (social structure). University of Wollongong, www.sociologydictionary.org/structure

Orme, J., Powell, J., Taylor, P., Harrison, T. and Grey, M. (2003) *Public Health for the 21st Century*. Buckingham, Cambridge University Press.

O'Sullivan, S. (2015) *It's All in Your Head: Stories from the Frontline of Psychosomatic Illness*. London, Vintage.

Patrick, R., Henderson-Wilson, C. and Ebden, M. (2021) Exploring the co-benefits of environmental volunteering for human and planetary health promotion. *Health Promot J of Australia,* 33, 57–67.

Pausé, C. (2018) Borderline: the ethics of fat stigma in public health. *Journal of Law, Medicine & Ethics,* 45, 510–17.

Pérez-Wilson, P., Marcos-Marcos, J., Morgan, A., Eriksson, M., Lindström, B. and Álvarez-Dardet, C. (2021) 'A synergy model of health': an integration of salutogenesis and the health assets model. *Health Promotion International,* 36, 844–94.

Perissinotto, C., Holt-Lunstad, Periyakoil, V.S. and Covinsky, K. (2019) A practical approach to assessing and mitigation loneliness and isolation in older adults. *Journal of the American Geriatrics Society,* 67 (4), 657–62.

Peterson, A., Davis, M., Fraser, S. and Lindsay, J. (2010) Healthy living and citizenship: an overview. *Critical Public Health,* 20, 391–400.

Phongsavan, P., Chey, T., Bauman, A., Brooks, R. and Silove, D. (2006) Social capital, socio-economic status and psychological distress among Australian adults. *Social Science & Medicine,* 63 (10), 2546–61.

Pickett, K. and Wilkinson, R. (2015) Income inequality and health: a causal review. *Soc Sci Med,* 128, 316–26.

Planès, S., Villier, C. and Mallaret, M. (2016) The nocebo effect of drugs. *Pharmacol Res Perspect,* 4 (2), doi:10.1002/prp2.208

Porter, R. (2020) The biopsychosocial model in mental health. *Australian & New Zealand Journal of Psychiatry,* 54 (8), doi:10.1177/0004867420944464

Prince, M., Patel, V., Saena, S., Maj, M., Maselko, J., Phillips, M.R. and Rahman, A. (2007) No health without mental health. *The Lancet,* 370 (9590), 8–14.

Rafique, M.Z., Sun, J., Larik, A.R. and Li, Y. (2022) Assessment of willingness to pay for pollution prevention, health and happiness: a case study of Punjab, Pakistan. *Frontiers in Public Health,* 10, doi:10.3389/fpubh.2022.825387

Ramos M.C., Cheng, C.E.., Preston, K.S.J., Gottfried, A.W., Guerin, D.W., Gottfried, A.E. et al. (2022) Positive family relationships across 30 years: predicting adult health and happiness. *Journal of Family Psychology,* 36 (7), 1216–28.

Ristovski-Slijepcevic, S., Bell, K., Chapman, G.E. and Beagan, B.L. (2010) Being 'thick' indicates you are eating, you are healthy and you have an attractive body shape: perspectives on fatness and food choice amongst Black and White men and women in Canada. *Health Sociology Review,* 19 (3), 317–29.

Röhrich, C., Giordano, J. and Kohls, N.B. (2021) Narrative view of the role of health promotion and salutogenesis in the treatment of chronic disease: viability and value for the care of cardiovascular conditions. *Cardiovascular Diagnosis and Therapy,* 11 (2), 591–601.

Rosen, A.O., Holmes, A.L., Balluerka, N., Hidalgo, M.D., Gorostiaga, A., Gómez-Benito et al. (2022) Is social media a new type of social support? Social media use in Spain during the COVID-19 pandemic: a mixed methods study. *Int J Environ Res Public Health,* 19 (7), doi:10.3390/ijerph19073952

Roy, S.C. (2008) 'Taking charge of your health': discourses of responsibility in English Canadian women's magazines. *Sociology of Health & Illness,* 30, 463–77.

Ruch, W. (2014) Cheerfulness. In Michalos, A.C. (ed.) *Encyclopedia of Quality of Life and Well-being Research,* Dordrecht, Springer.

Saracci, R. (1997) The World Health Organization needs to reconsider its definition of health. *BMJ,* 314: 1409, doi:10.1136/bmj.314.7091.1409

Sarafino, E.P. and Smith, T.W. (2022) *Health Psychology: Biopsychosocial Interactions.* 10th edition. Chichester, Wiley.

Sartorius, N. (2006) The meanings of health and its promotion. *Croatian Medical Journal,* 47 (4), 662–4.

Savage, M., Devine, F., Cunningham, N., Taylor, M., Li, Y., Hjellbrekke, J. et al. (2013) A new model of social class? Findings from the BBC's Great British Class Survey experiment. *Sociology,* 47, 219–50.

Savila, F., Leakehe, P., Bagg, W., Harwood, M., Letele, D., Bamber, A. et al. (2022) Understanding engagement with Brown Buttabean Motivation, an Auckland grassroots, Pacific-led holistic health programme: a qualitative study. *BMJ Open,* 12, doi:10.1136/bmjopen-2021-059854

Schoon, P.M. and Krumwiede, K. (2022) A holistic health determinants model for public health nursing education and practice. *Public Health Nursing,* 39, 1070–7.

Scriven, A. (2017) *Ewles and Simnett's Promoting Health: A Practical Guide.* 7th edition. London, Elsevier.

Seedhouse, D. (2001) *Health: The Foundations for Achievement.* 2nd edition. Chichester, Wiley.

Seligman, M. (2011) *Flourish.* New York: Free Press.

Seligman, M. (2018) PERMA and the building blocks of wellbeing. *Journal of Positive Psychology,* 13 (4), 333–5.

Shome, D., Vadera, S., Optom, S.R.M.O. and Kapoor, R. (2020) Does taking selfies lead to increased desire to undergo cosmetic surgery? *J Cosmet Dermatol,*19, 2025–32.

Sidell, M. (2010) Older People's Health: Applying Antonovsky's Salutogenic Paradigm. In Douglas, J., Earle, S., Handsley, L.,

Jones, L., Lloyd, C. and Spurr, S. (eds.) *A Reader in Promoting Public Health: Challenges and Controversy.* 2nd edition. London, Sage.

Skovdal, M. (2013) Using Theory to Guide Change at the Community Level. In Cragg, L., Davis, M. and Macdowall, W. (eds.) *Health Promotion Theory.* 2nd edition. Maidenhead, Open University Press.

Smith, L. and Nersesian, P. (2024) Reimagining Child and Family Health Education and Health Promotion through a Planetary Health Lens. In Cross, R. (ed.) *Health Promotion and Health Education for Nurses.* London, Sage.

Smylie, J. and Anderson, M. (2006) Understanding the health of Indigenous peoples in Canada: key methodological and conceptual challenges. *CMAJ,* 175 (6), 602–6.

Solar, O. and Irwin, A. (2010) *A Conceptual Framework for Action on the Social Determinants of Health.* Social Determinants of Health Discussion Paper 2 (Policy and Practice). Geneva, World Health Organization.

Stainton-Rogers, W. (1991) *Explaining Health and Illness: An Exploration of Diversity.* London, Harvester Wheatsheaf.

Steckermeier, L.C. and Delhey, J. (2019) Better for everyone? Egalitarian culture and social wellbeing in Europe. *Social Indicators Research,* 143, 1075–108.

Steptoe, A. (2019) Happiness and health. *Annual Review of Public Health,* 40, 339–59.

Stevens, A. and Griffiths, S. (2020) Body positivity (#BoPo) in everyday life: an ecological momentary assessment study showing potential benefits to individuals' body image and emotional wellbeing. *Body Image,* 35, 181–91.

Stoewen, D.L. (2017) Dimensions of wellness: change your habits, change your life. *Veterinary Wellness,* 58, 861–2.

Stokes, K., Noren, J. and Shindell, S. (1982) Definition of terms and concepts applicable to clinical preventive medicine. *Journal of Community Health,* 8 (1), 33–41.

Sujarwoto, S. (2021) Does happiness pays? A longitudinal family life survey. *Applied Research in Quality of Life,* 16 (2), 679–701.

Sun, J. and Yang, K. (2016) The wicked problem of climate change: a new approach based on social mess and fragmentation. *Sustainability,* 8 (12), doi:10.3390/su8121312

Svalastog, A.L., Donev, D., Kristoffersen, J. and Gajovíc, S. (2017) Concepts and definitions of health and health-related values in the knowledge landscapes of the digital society. *Croatian Medical Journal,* 58, 431–5.

Tapper, K. (2021) *Health Psychology and Behaviour Change.* London, Red Globe Press.

Taylor, J., O'Hara, L. and Barnes, M. (2014) Health promotion: a critical salutogenic science. *International Journal of Social Work and Human Services Practice,* 2 (6), 283–90.

Tedeschi, B. (2017) Where a doctor saw treatable cancer, a patient saw an evil spirit, https://www.statnews.com/2017/06/30/hmong -cancer-doctor-patient

Tennant, R., Hiller, L., Fishwick, R., Platt, S., Joseph, S., Wiech, S. et al. (2007) The Warwick-Edinburgh Mental Wellbeing Scale (WEMWBS): development and UK validation. *Health and Quality of Life Outcomes,* 5 (63), doi:10.1186/1477-7525-5-63

Theofilou, P. (2013) Quality of life: definition and measurement. *Europe's Journal of Psychology,* 9 (1), 150–62.

Tomlinson, M.W. and Kelly, G.P. (2013) Is everybody happy? The politics and measurement of national wellbeing. *Policy & Politics,* 41 (2), 139–57.

Tranter, H., Brooks, M. and Khan, R. (2021) Emotional resilience and event centrality mediate posttraumatic growth following adverse childhood experiences. *Psychological Trauma: Theory, Research, Practice, and Policy,* 13 (2), 165–73.

Tremblay, M. and Martin, D.H. (2023) Etuaptmumk/Two-Eyed Seeing: A Guiding Principle to Respectfully *Embrace* Indigenous and Western Systems of Knowledge. In Jourdan, D. and Potvin, L. (eds.) *Global Handbook for Health Promotion Research, Vol. 3: Doing Health Promotion Research.* Cham: Springer.

Tremblay, S.C., Tremblay, S.E. and Poirier, P. (2021) From filters to fillers: an action inference approach to body image distortion in the selfie era. *AI & Society,* 36, 33–48.

Trudel-Fitzgerald, C., James, P., Kim, E.S., Zevon, E.S., Grodstein, F. and Kubzansky, L.D. (2019) Prospective associations of happiness and optimism with lifestyle over up to two decades. *Preventive Medicine,* 126, doi:10.1016/j.ypmed.2019.105754

Tsuruta, K., Shiomitsu, T., Hombu, A. and Fujii, Y. (2019) Relationship between social capital and happiness in a Japanese community: a cross-sectional study. *Nursing & Health Sciences,* 21, 245–52.

Turrentine, J. (2022) What are the causes of climate change? NRDC, www.nrdc.org/stories/what-are-causes-climate-change #natural

UNDRR (United Nations Office for Disaster Risk Reduction) (2022) Underlying disaster risk drivers, https://www.undrr.org /terminology/underlying-disaster-risk-drivers

United Nations (1986) Declaration on the Right to Development, https://www.ohchr.org/en/documents/instruments/declaration -right-development

United Nations (2022) Population, www.un.org/en/global-issues /population

United Nations Population Division (2023) Life expectancy of the world population, www.worldmeters.info/demographics/life -expectancy

Universal Declaration of Human Rights (1948), https://www.un.org /en/about-us/universal-declaration-of-human-rights

van den Eijnden, R.J.J.M., Lemmens, J.S. and Valkenburg, P.M. (2016) The social media disorder scale. *Computers in Human Behavior,* 61, 478–87.

Vassallo, A., Jones, A. and Freeman, B. (2021) Social media: frenemy of public health? *Public Health Nutrition,* doi:10.1017 /S136898002100269X

Veehoven, R. (2003) Hedonism and happiness. *Journal of Happiness Studies: An Interdisciplinary Forum on Subjective Well-Being,* 4 (4), 437–57.

Veiga, G.R.S., Padilha, B.M., Bueno, N.B., Santos, J.R.L., Nunes, L.F., Florencio, T.M.T. and Lima, M.C. (2022) Salutogenesis, nutritional status and eating behaviour: a systematic review. *Public Health Nutrition,* 25 (9), 2517–29.

Vendemia, M.A. and Robinson, M.J. (2022) Promoting body positivity through stories: how protagonist body size and esteem influence readers' self-concepts. *Body Image,* 42, 315–16.

Vizheh, M., Qorbani, M., Arzaghi, S.M., Muhidin, S., Javanmard, Z. and Esmaeili, M. (2020) The mental health of healthcare workers in the COVID-19 pandemic: a systematic review. *Journal of Diabetes & Metabolic Disorders,* 19, 1967–78.

Walls, H. (2018) Wicked problems and a 'wicked' solution. *Globalization and Health,* 14 (34), doi:10.1186/s12992-018 -0353-x

Walls, M., Hautala, D., Cole, A., Kosobuski, L., Weiss, N., Hill, K. et al. (2022) Socio-cultural integration and holistic health among Indigenous young adults. *BMC Public Health,* 22, doi:10.1186 /s12889-022-13395-3

Wang, Q., Zhao, X., Yuan, Y. and Shi, B. (2021) The relationship between creativity and intrusive rumination among Chinese teenagers during the COVID-19 pandemic: emotional resilience as a moderator. *Front. Psychol.,* 11, doi:10.3389/fpsyg.2020 .601104

Wang, W., Sun, Y., Chen, Y. Bu, Y and Li, G. (2022) Health effects of happiness in China. *Int J Environ Res Public Health,* 19, doi:10.3390/ijerph19116686

Ward, M., McGarrigle, C.A. and Kenny, R.A. (2019) More than health: quality of life trajectories among older adults – findings from the Irish Longitudinal Study of Ageing (TILDA). *Quality of Life Research,* 28, 429–39.

Warwick-Booth, L. and Cross, R. (2018) *Global Health Studies: A Social Determinants Perspective.* Cambridge, Polity.

Warwick-Booth, L., Cross, R. and Lowcock, D. (2021) *Contemporary Health Studies: An Introduction.* 2nd edition. Cambridge, Polity.

Wathne, K. (2014) *Obesity: Culture, Family, Individual. A Qualitative Study of Fat in Youth.* PhD thesis, University of Oslo, Norway.

Welsh, T. (2011) Healthism and the bodies of women: pleasure and discipline in the war against obesity. *Journal of Feminist Scholarship,* 1, 33–48.

White, A., McKee, M. Richardson, N., Madsen, S.A., de Sousa, B., de Visser, R. et al. (2017) Europe's men need their own health strategy. *British Medical Journal,* 343, d7397.

White, S.C. (2017) Relational wellbeing: re-centring the politics of happiness, policy and self. *Policy & Politics,* 45, 121–36.

Whitmarsh, L., Player, L., Jiongco, A., James, M., Williams, M., Marks, E., Kennedy-Williams, P. (2022), Climate anxiety: what predicts it and how is it related to climate action? *Journal of Environmental Psychology,* 83, 101866.

Whitmee, S. et al. (2015) Safeguarding human health in the Anthropocene epoch: report of the Rockefeller Foundation – Lancet Commission on planetary health. *The Lancet,* 386 (10007), 1973–2028.

Wilkinson, I. (2006) Psychology and Risk. In Mythen, G. and Walklate, S. (eds.) *Beyond the Risk Society: Critical Reflections on Risk and Human Society.* Maidenhead, Open University Press.

Wilkinson, R. and Pickett, K. (2009) *The Spirit Level: Why More Equal Societies Almost Always Do Better.* London, Penguin.

Wilkinson, R. and Pickett, K. (2018) *The Inner Level: How More Equal Societies Reduce Stress, Restore Sanity and Improve Everyone's Well-being.* London, Penguin.

Williams, E., Buck, D., Babalola, G. and Maguire, D. (2022) *What Are Health Inequalities?* The King's Fund, www.kingsfund.org .uk/publications/what-are-health-inequalities

Williams, L. and Mumtaz, Z. (2007) *Being Alive Well: Aboriginal Youth and Evidenced-Based Approaches to Promoting Wellbeing,* http://www.researchgate.net/publication/263426532

Williams, P. (2022) Climate anxiety: what predicts it and how is it related to climate action? *Journal of Environmental Psychology,* 83, doi:10.1016/j.jenvp.2022.101866

Wills, J. (2023) *Foundations for Health Promotion*. 5th edition. London, Elsevier.

Wilson, D., Moloney, E., Parr, J.M., Aspinall, C. and Slark, J. (2021) Creating an Indigenous Māori-centred model of relational health: a literature review of Māori models of health. *Journal of Clinical Nursing*, 30, 3539–55.

Wind, T.R. and Villalonga-Olives, E. (2018) Social capital interventions in public health: moving towards why social capital matters for health. *J Epidemiology & Community Health*, 73 (9), doi:10.1136/jech-2018-211576

Wismar, M., Lahtinen, E., Ståhl, T., Ollila, E. and Leppo, K. (2018) Introduction. In Ståhl, T., Wismar, M., Ollila, E., Lahtinen, E. and Leppo, K. (eds.) *Health in All Policies: Prospects and Potentials*. Finland, European Observatory on Health Systems and Policies.

Woodall, J. and Cross, R. (2022) *Essentials of Health Promotion*. London, Sage.

World Bank (2023) Life expectancy at birth, total (years), https://data.worldbank.org/indicator/SP.DYN.LE00.IN

World Economic Forum (2015) How should we measure wellbeing?, https://www.weforum.org/agenda/2015/01/how-should-we-measure-wellbeing-2

World Health Organization (1986) The Ottawa Charter, https://intranet.euro.who.int/__data/assets/pdf_file/0004/129532/Ottawa_Charter.pdf

World Health Organization (2006a) The definition of health, https://www.who.int/teams/sexual-and-reproductive-health-and-research-(srh)/areas-of-work/sexual-health

World Health Organization (2006b) *Defining Sexual Health: A Report of a Technical Consultation on Sexual Health, 28–31 January, 2002*. Geneva, WHO.

World Health Organization (2008) *The Right to Health*. Fact Sheet 31. Geneva, WHO.

World Health Organization (2009) Mental Health, https://www.who.int/news-room/fact-sheets/detail/mental-health-strengthening-our-response

World Health Organization (2014) Mental health: a state of wellbeing, www.who.int/features/factfiles/mental_health/en

World Health Organization (2017) One Health, www.who.int/news-room/questions-and-answers/item/one-health

World Health Organization (2021) The Geneva Charter for Well-being, https://www.who.int/publications/m/item/the-geneva-charter-for-well-being

World Health Organization (2022) *World Mental Health Report: Transforming Mental Health for All*. Geneva, WHO.

World Health Organization (2023) Constitution of the World Health Organization, https://www.who.int/about/accountability/governance/constitution

World Population Review (2023) Happiest countries in the world 2023, worldpopulationreview.com

Wynes, S. and Nicholas, K.A. (2017) The climate mitigation gap: education and government recommendations miss the most effective individual actions. *Environmental Research Letters,* 12 (7), doi:10.1088/1748-9326/aa7541

Yang, S. Dingfang, S. and Yin, H. (2022) 'Teaching, my passion; publishing, my pain': unpacking academics' professional identity tensions through the lens of emotional resilience. *Higher Education,* 84, 235–54.

Yang, Y., Bekemeier, B. and Choi, J. (2018) A cultural and contextual analysis of health concepts and needs of women in a rural district of Nepal. *Global Health Promotion,* 25 (1), 15–22.

Yuan, M., Yue-qun, C., Wang, H. and Hong, X. (2021) Does social capital promote health? *Social Indicators Research,* 162, 501–24.

Zhang, J., Marino, C., Canale, N., Charrier, L., Lazzeri, G., Nardone, P. and Vieno, A. (2022a) The effect of problematic social media use on happiness among adolescents: the mediating role of lifestyle habits. *Int J Environ Res Public Health,* 19 (5), doi:10.3390/ijerph19052576

Zhang, J.H., Ramke, J., Jan, C., Bascaran, C., Mwangi, N., Furtado, J.M. et al. (2022b) Advancing the Sustainable Development Goals through improving eye health: a scoping review. *Lancet Planet Health,* 6, e270–80.

Zhang, R., Tang, X., Liu, J., Visbeck, M., Guo, H., Murray, V. et al. (2022c) From concept to action: a united, holistic and One Health approach to respond to the climate change crisis. *Infectious Diseases of Poverty,* 11 (17), doi:10.1186/s40249-022-00941-9

Ziglio, E., Azzopardi-Muscat, N. and Briguglio, L. (2017) Resilience and 21st century public health. *European Journal of Public Health,* 27 (5), 789–90.

Index

Page numbers in **bold type** refer to a table or figure.